How to Lower Your Blood Pressure

Christine Craggs-Hinton, mother of three, followed a career in the civil service until, in 1991, she developed fibromyalgia, a chronic pain condition. Christine took up writing for therapeutic reasons, and has in the past few years produced more than a dozen books for Sheldon Press, including *Living with Fibromyalgia*, *The Chronic Fatigue Healing Diet*, *Coping Successfully with Psoriasis* and *How to Manage Chronic Fatigue*. Since moving to the Canary Islands, where she is the resident agony aunt for a local newspaper, she has also taken up fiction writing.

Overcoming Common Problems Series

Selected titles

A full list of titles is available from Sheldon Press,
36 Causton Street, London SW1P 4ST and on our website at
www.sheldonpress.co.uk

Overcoming Common Problems

How to Lower Your Blood Pressure

And keep it down

CHRISTINE CRAGGS-HINTON

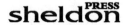
sheldon **PRESS**

First published in Great Britain in 2010

Sheldon Press
36 Causton Street
London SW1P 4ST
www.sheldonpress.co.uk

British Library Cataloguing-in-Publication Data
A catalogue record for this book is available from the British Library

ISBN 978-1-84709-095-9

1 3 5 7 9 10 8 6 4 2

Typeset by Fakenham Photosetting Ltd, Fakenham, Norfolk
Printed in Great Britain by Ashford Colour Press

Produced on paper from sustainable forests

Contents

Author's note to the reader

This book is intended as a guide to help you lower diagnosed high blood pressure – often in combination with prescribed medications. It is not a medical book and it is not intended to replace advice from your doctor. If you think you have high blood pressure and have not yet consulted your doctor, please do so.

Introduction

High blood pressure is a common condition in Westernized countries, particularly among the elderly. In non-Westernized countries, where people are more physically active, eat plenty of fruit, vegetables and grain and have a low salt and alcohol intake, high blood pressure is rare, even in the elderly. It is not an inevitable consequence of getting older, as many people think; rather, it is usually a result of a few lifestyle factors. Of course, high blood pressure can also run in the family, which means there is sometimes a genetic component.

Unfortunately, a person with high blood pressure stands a greater chance of developing cardiovascular (heart) disease, stroke, kidney disease or impaired vision than a person with normal blood pressure. High blood pressure seldom gives rise to symptoms, however – which are the body's warning mechanism that something is wrong. This means the condition can go undetected for years or even decades. In the meantime, the problems related to high blood pressure will invariably progress and become more serious. For many, it's not until a health emergency takes them to the accident and emergency department of their local hospital that their high blood pressure is detected. That's why getting your blood pressure checked on a regular basis is so important, especially if you belong to a high risk group, such as having a parent with high blood pressure, or if you live on your nerves and smoke cigarettes. The typical high blood pressure candidate is overweight, sedentary, over 60 and a smoker. He or she may already have high cholesterol or even diabetes. There are plenty of other people with high blood pressure who don't fit this model at all, however, which makes it doubly important that every one of us undergoes regular blood pressure screening.

High blood pressure is on the increase and in the next few years is expected to rise by approximately 25 per cent in Westernized countries, affecting one in three of the adult population. Currently, one in four adults in the West have high blood pressure. In the UK, around 50 per cent of people over 65 have it, as have some 70 per cent of those in their 70s. These figures are truly staggering when you consider that high blood pressure is very easy to diagnose and treat. Indeed, the condition is one of the most preventable causes of death in the developed world.

In the UK, high blood pressure has become the second most common reason for a person to visit his or her doctor. That said, statisticians believe the condition is only adequately treated in one-fifth of cases. Even more shocking is the estimation that 35 per cent of people with high blood pressure are unaware that they have it.

High blood pressure usually lasts a lifetime, but can be effectively lowered to within the healthy range. Public awareness of the dangers of high blood pressure is greater now than ever before, which means that more and more people are likely to know that they are in a high risk category and will therefore ask to have their blood pressure checked by their doctor. There are still plenty of people diagnosed with high blood pressure who remain ignorant to its dangers and so fail to make essential lifestyle adjustments or even bother to take their medication on a daily basis. Don't let this happen to you! Arm yourself with knowledge and take all the practical steps required to improve your future. Lifestyle modifications – and blood pressure medications, if necessary – can be of enormous benefit, for they slow down the progression of cardiovascular (heart) disease. They also reduce the risk of stroke and many more dangers.

This book looks at how you can lower your blood pressure by making changes to your lifestyle. It also acknowledges that blood pressure drugs may have a vital part to play. Topics include:

- the dangers of high blood pressure
- a healthy diet and reducing obesity
- the importance of exercise and how to choose an exercise regime
- managing stress
- quitting smoking
- women and high blood pressure
- blood pressure medication
- complementary remedies.

1

High blood pressure – an overview

Blood is carried to all the tissues and organs in the body through a network of tubes called *arteries*, having been given a strong 'push' by the heart, which acts as a pump. The heart normally beats approximately 60–70 times a minute, pumping out blood in which fluids and nutrients are carried around the body. The term *blood pressure* is the measurement of the force of blood as it rushes through the arteries.

When blood pressure is categorized as 'high' – a condition known as *hypertension* – the pressure of blood in the arteries is consistently greater than it should be, exerting tremendous force against the arterial walls. This puts these small vessels – which may already be narrow or rigid owing to genetic factors (see below) – under a lot of strain. In time, untreated high blood pressure is likely to damage the arteries and cause heart abnormalities. High blood pressure is, in fact, one of the main risk factors for developing cardiovascular disease, which means disease of the heart and arteries.

There are two numbers that make up a blood pressure reading – a higher one and a lower one. As the force of blood is greatest when the heart contracts to push blood through the arteries, this is the higher of the two numbers and is known as the systolic pressure. The lower of the two numbers relates to when the heart is momentarily at rest between beats and is known as diastolic pressure (see Figures 1 and 2 overleaf).

The two numbers are usually written down with the higher number (systolic pressure) on top or slightly to the left of the lower number (diastolic pressure) – e.g. 120/80. A person will normally refer to a blood pressure reading as '120 over 80', or whatever the two numbers are. Systolic pressure can sit anywhere between 90 and 240, and diastolic pressure can sit anywhere between 60 and 140. A blood pressure reading of below 120/80 is considered normal. To be more accurate, though, the systolic blood pressure in a healthy individual

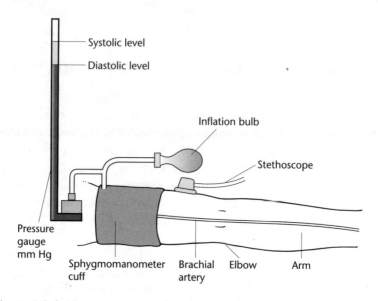

Figure 1 Sphygmomanometer showing pressure gauge

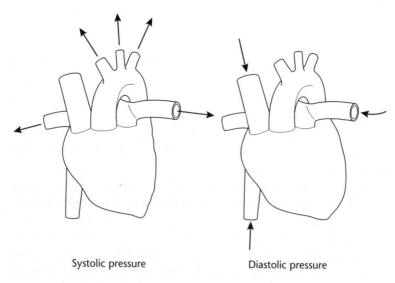

Systolic pressure   Diastolic pressure

Figure 2 Systolic and diastolic pressure
Arrows show direction of blood flow

should measure between 90 and 120, and the diastolic pressure should measure between 60 and 80.

With each heartbeat, a person's blood pressure rises and falls between the two numbers, and as blood pressure is measured in units called millimetres of mercury – expressed as *mm Hg* – you will often see 'mm Hg' written down after the two numbers.

We all have a different blood pressure and it can change throughout the day. It is usually at its lowest during sleep and rises as you get up in the morning. It can also rise when you are excited, stressed or being unusually active.

Although high blood pressure is a serious condition, it is not generally accompanied by symptoms and can exist for many years without you being aware of it. Indeed, the serious complications which can build up over time have led to the condition being dubbed 'the silent killer' – and the higher the blood pressure, the greater the risk of serious, even fatal, complications. For most people, it is only possible to know whether or not you have high blood pressure by having it checked. Most doctors will take their patients' blood pressure every three to five years, and more frequently as they get older. Individuals with a previous high reading should have their blood pressure checked on a regular basis.

There are two types of high blood pressure – *essential* and *secondary* hypertension. In the majority of cases of essential hypertension, the blood vessels (arteries, veins and capillaries) that are most distant from the heart become narrow or hard over time, which causes the pressure of blood to build up. Essential hypertension (sometimes referred to as *primary* hypertension) accounts for about 95 per cent of cases and often runs in families, which means the cause is genetic. Indeed, if you have a parent with high blood pressure you stand a fair chance of getting it yourself. If both parents have high blood pressure, you are twice as likely to develop it. Also, you are more likely to develop high blood pressure early if that's what happened to your parent. Although the genes that make a person prone to developing high blood pressure have not yet been identified, researchers are looking at the genetic factors involved in blood pressure regulation – i.e. salt balance and arterial elasticity.

Essential hypertension is more often linked to lack of exercise, being overweight, excessive salt intake, ageing and genetics than to secondary hypertension. There is also more likelihood of arterial stiffness.

Secondary hypertension accounts for only about 5 per cent of all high blood pressure cases and refers to high blood pressure that is caused by (or secondary to) a specific abnormality in one of the organs or systems of the body – i.e. diabetes or kidney disease. It has been estimated that about three out of ten people with Type 1 diabetes and more than half of people with Type 2 diabetes go on to develop high blood pressure. If you have diabetes, your doctor will tell you which type you have.

In the UK, it's estimated that about 50 per cent of people over the age of 65 have high blood pressure, as have about one in four middle-aged adults. Most cases are mildly high (with a reading of up to 160/100), but more than one in 20 adults have blood pressure in excess of 160/100. High blood pressure is far less common in younger adults.

How is high blood pressure defined?

High blood pressure is defined as the following:

- A consistent systolic (the number on top) blood pressure reading of 140 or more. The systolic reading indicates the pressure of blood against arterial walls.
- And/or a diastolic (the number on the bottom) blood pressure reading of 90 or more. The diastolic reading indicates the pressure in the arteries while the heart is filling and resting between beats.

If your blood pressure reading is between 120/80 and 140/90 it is classified by doctors as *prehypertension*, meaning above normal but not in the level considered to be 'high'. Readings of 131/83, 122/89 and 139/86 are in the normal or prehypertension range. For people with such readings, changing your lifestyle can put you out of danger, whereas continuing to pursue habits such as smoking, eating a lot of salt, drinking alcohol to excess, and so on, can easily push you into the high blood pressure range.

A blood pressure measuring 140/90 or more is classed as high blood pressure and your levels will require regular monitoring over a period of time. In some individuals it's possible for a high reading to be a 'one-off' – for instance, your car broke down so you had to hurry a long way on foot to the health centre, feeling flustered because you knew you were late. Frequent blood pressure monitoring, perhaps at different times of the day, is therefore essential. If the reading remains high, your doctor will want to monitor it regularly.

High blood pressure is a serious condition. To reduce the risk of serious health consequences, it is important that it is tackled from as many angles as possible. A variety of lifestyle changes can be of great benefit, all of which are mentioned in this book. However, some people will need to take medication, too.

It is possible to have a raised diastolic pressure but normal systolic pressure, and vice versa. However, in the majority of cases both pressures are raised.

Categories of high blood pressure

Although both the systolic and diastolic readings are important, a rise in diastolic pressure is more serious than a rise in systolic pressure. Indeed, whether a person is classed as mildly, moderately or severely affected is usually dependent upon the diastolic reading (see Table 1).

Table 1 Categories of high blood pressure

Diastolic pressure	Mildly affected	Moderately affected	Severely affected
90–104	√		
105–114		√	
115 or above			√

It should be said that in a small number of people, the systolic reading is abnormally high while the diastolic reading is within the normal range. For example, a reading of 160/80 is classed as high blood pressure in the moderate range, and 145/77 is classed as high blood pressure in the mild range.

When blood pressure is very high

A small percentage of people with high blood pressure do have symptoms – and it's almost always when the reading is extremely high. Symptoms include severe headaches, dizziness, blurred vision and nausea. If you have not yet had your blood pressure checked but have been experiencing the above symptoms, you should see your doctor as a matter of urgency. Your blood pressure may already be dangerously high, the diastolic figure possibly around the 140 mark, which is almost double the norm. With a reading so high, immediate hospitalization is necessary to prevent a brain haemorrhage or a stroke.

How is blood pressure measured?

Blood pressure can be measured by means of the more old-fashioned aneroid sphygmomanometer apparatus or the newer digital monitor. These devices look and work very differently:

- The sphygmomanometer apparatus comprises a mercury pressure gauge and an inflatable rubber or nylon cuff, which wraps around the person's arm and is inflated with an air pump to a pressure at which the flow of blood in the main artery (*brachial artery*) in the arm is blocked off (see Figures 3 and 4). As a result, the pulse at the elbow cannot be detected with a stethoscope. Now the cuff on the artery is gradually released and the reading at which the doctor or nurse first hears a pulsation from the artery is the systolic pressure (when the heart is contracting). Further pressure is released from the cuff and the pressure at which the pulsation eventually stops is the diastolic pressure (when the heart is resting between contractions). The sphygmomanometer is being used less and less often, owing to its bulk and frequent inaccurate measurements. *Sphygmo* is the Greek word for 'pulse' and a *manometer* is an apparatus for measuring pressure.
- Although most GPs still use aneroid sphygmomanometers, there is a variety of digital blood pressure monitors on the market, for home use (see Figure 5 overleaf). However, these devices are not always as accurate as the sphygmomanometer and in many

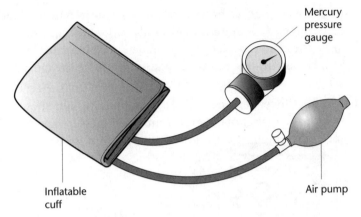

Mercury
pressure
gauge

Inflatable
cuff

Air pump

Figure 3 Aneroid sphygmomanometer

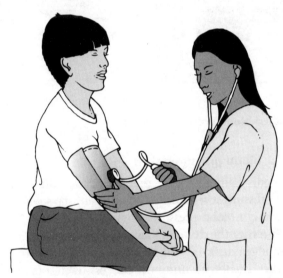

Figure 4 Doctor using aneroid sphygmomanometer on patient

cases will just give the user a rough idea of his or her blood pressure reading. As part of the monitoring process, some GPs will ask a patient with suspected high blood pressure to use a digital device between visits to the medical centre. Digital blood pressure monitors are portable and therefore much smaller than the sphygmomanometer. A digital monitor will comprise a cuff which wraps around the wrist. The individual sits up straight with the wrist cuff at heart level. A 'start–stop' button should now be pressed to automatically inflate the cuff and digitally display the reading. The digital models recommended by the British Hypertension Society are considered to be the most accurate when used properly. (See the 'Useful addresses' section on p. 113 for details of this society.)

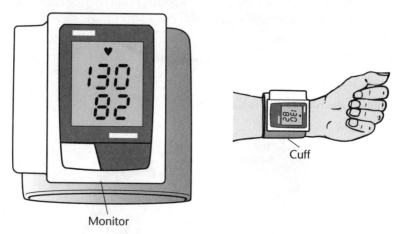

Monitor

Cuff

Figure 5 Digital blood pressure monitor

Having your blood pressure taken

As mentioned, your doctor or practice nurse will want to take your blood pressure several times on different days before giving a diagnosis of high blood pressure. Having it checked is simple and quick, using either the more old-fashioned sphygmomanometer or the more modern digital blood pressure monitor. You will be asked to either sit or lie down during the process, which takes only two or three minutes in all.

Here are a few things you can do beforehand:

- Avoid drinking coffee or smoking cigarettes 30 minutes prior to having your blood pressure taken.
- Go to the toilet before the reading, as a full bladder can change the reading slightly.
- Wear short sleeves.
- Sit and relax for five minutes before the reading.

Afterwards, ask for your blood pressure reading in numbers – i.e. in the form '135 over 95'.

Using a digital monitor at home

If you would like to check your blood pressure at home between medical appointments, it's best to ask your doctor, nurse or pharmacist to show you how to use the monitor properly (see Figure 6).

The following pointers should also help:

- Sit with your back supported and your feet flat on the floor.
- Rest your arm on a table at the level of your heart (you may need to place your arm on a cushion to achieve the correct height).
- Take three readings several minutes apart. Your true result is the average of all three.
- Try to take your blood pressure at the same time every day, such as one hour after eating breakfast, before any strenuous exercise, before smoking and prior to any caffeine intake.
- If your blood pressure appears to be high or even borderline, it's important that you have it checked by your doctor as soon as possible.

Blood pressure machines in supermarkets and pharmacies

You have probably noticed that many supermarkets and pharmacies now have blood pressure machines. So, are they accurate? Well, according to a recent study, they are usually accurate but occasionally not. Unfortunately, it's not normally possible to tell whether or not they are working properly, even if the cuff fits snugly around your arm and self-inflates. Obviously, if the cuff doesn't fit properly and/or self-inflate, the machine isn't working properly.

You should be careful to use the machine as directed.

Don't rely on the reading from one machine

Please note that relying solely on home digital monitors and machines in supermarkets and pharmacies is not a good idea. They're excellent for giving you an indication of your blood pressure level, but it's important also to have your blood pressure regularly checked by a doctor or nurse with an accurate device.

White coat hypertension

Some people experience high blood pressure in their doctor's surgery and not in normal situations – a phenomenon known as *white coat hypertension*. Such people are also liable to a rise in blood pressure when faced with an authority figure of some kind. In some cases, the officious manner with which they are dealt is the problem, whereas in others it seems that the problem is anxiety over what they are about to be told. White coat hypertension is, therefore, an artificial reading. A diagnosis of white coat hypertension is not a clinically important finding.

One in four people who are diagnosed with mild high blood pressure actually have normal blood pressure when away from the anxiety and stress of their doctor's surgery. To avoid giving a wrong diagnosis, your doctor should fit you with an *ambulatory* monitor so that your blood pressure away from the doctor's surgery can be taken. The device is normally worn for 24 hours and automatically takes your blood pressure every 30 minutes.

A family history of high blood pressure

Scientists recently determined that 39 per cent of male African Americans and 43 per cent of female African Americans have high blood pressure – figures that are far higher than in the remainder of the US population. Therefore, high blood pressure clearly has a genetic component. This fact was demonstrated when, in July 2009, researchers reported the discovery of five defective (*rogue*) genes linked to high blood pressure in African Americans. In that same year, researchers found a massive 13 rogue genes related to high blood pressure in people of European and South Asian ancestry. Each genetic defect is associated with only a slight increase in blood pressure – however, the researchers were able to prove that the more defects in existence, the more likelihood there was of high blood pressure occurring. One of these genes is already targeted in an existing class of drug called *calcium channel-blockers* (see Chapter 7).

In due course, researchers should be able to find more genes associated with blood pressure. This should help them to develop improved treatment options for the millions of people affected.

Researchers are also attempting to identify blood-pressure-related genetic anomalies in other societies of people.

Other risk factors for developing high blood pressure

It's not possible to change our genes or the fact that we age with time – both of which can influence whether or not we develop high blood pressure. However, blood pressure also reacts greatly to the way we live our lives. It is therefore possible to improve your blood pressure by changing your lifestyle.

The following are lifestyle risk factors for developing high blood pressure:

- being overweight
- smoking
- not taking enough exercise
- enduring long-lasting stress
- drinking excess alcohol
- high salt intake
- not getting enough potassium in your diet
- eating an unhealthy high fat, high carbohydrate diet
- drinking a lot of coffee or other caffeine-rich drinks.

If you can identify more than one of the above risk factors in your own lifestyle, you are increasing your risk of developing high blood pressure. In addition, many risk factors react with each other, which also increases the risk. For example, a middle-aged smoker who lives a sedentary lifestyle and has high blood pressure stands a far greater chance of having a heart attack before the age of 60 than a middle-aged non-smoker who takes plenty of exercise.

Whether you already have high blood pressure or are in a high risk group and want to prevent its onset, it's vitally important that you make lifestyle changes wherever you can. For instance, if you are overweight and sit at a desk all day and in front of the TV for most of the night, you can improve your diet and become more active. If you smoke and have a lot of salt in your diet, you can quit smoking and cut down on the salt. (See Chapters 2, 3, 4 and 5 for more information on how to change your lifestyle so that you are more able to control your blood pressure.)

Fixed risk factors

Unfortunately, there are also risk factors that are impossible to alter, such as whether or not high blood pressure runs in your family (see below). Such risk factors include the following:

- *Your family history (genes)* For example, your risk is greater if you have a father or brother who developed cardiovascular disease or suffered a stroke before the age of 55, or a mother or sister before the age of 65.
- *Age* For example, the older you grow the more likely you are to develop degeneration of the arterial walls, causing restricted blood circulation and therefore high blood pressure.
- *Your ethnic group* For example, people living in the UK but with an ancestry from India, Bangladesh, Pakistan or Sri Lanka are known to stand a greater risk than Caucasians of developing high blood pressure. The same is the case with African Americans and people of Afro-Caribbean origin. People in these groups are also more likely to develop high blood pressure at an earlier age than Caucasians.
- *Your socio-economic status* For example, high blood pressure is more common in poorly educated and lower socio-economic groups.

Owing to the protective effects of oestrogen, the female hormone, it was always believed that women were less likely than men to develop high blood pressure. Experts have now concluded that while statistically this is true (statistics work in a complicated way), when everything is taken into account both sexes are at similar risk. The reason for this is that for women unique factors can cause their blood pressure to rise, such as use of the contraceptive pill, pregnancy, the menopause and use of hormone replacement therapy (HRT).

For more in-depth information on women and high blood pressure, see Chapter 8.

Treatable risk factors

Treatable or partly treatable risk factors include:

- diabetes (Type 1 and Type 2)

- kidney diseases and other problems that affect kidney function
- high cholesterol blood level
- high triglyceride blood level – triglycerides are a product of natural fats and oils
- thyroid dysfunction
- taking certain medicines
- tumours or other unusual genetic disorders which affect the hormones produced by the adrenal glands.

If any of these apply to you and you also have high blood pressure, it is more important than ever that you and your doctor work together to get your blood pressure under control.

As mentioned, taking certain medicines can cause high blood pressure. These include amphetamines (stimulants), the birth control pill, diet pills and some pills used for treating colds and allergies. If you are taking any of these medications and have high blood pressure, it's worth asking your doctor if you can change to another type of medication which treats the same problem. Your blood pressure may respond by going down.

Possible complications of high blood pressure

When high blood pressure is untreated – either because it is not discovered or because you fail to take steps to control it – your heart has to work much harder than it should, your arteries take a hammering and you are at great risk of the condition progressing and eventually damaging critical organs, with potentially fatal consequences.

The possible complications are as shown below and in Figure 6:

- Small swellings called *aneurisms* may develop in arterial walls. Common locations for these are in the aorta (the main artery carrying blood from the heart) and arteries in the brain, legs, spleen and intestines.
- Early hardening of the arteries (known as *arteriosclerosis*) can occur throughout the body, particularly in the heart, brain, kidneys and legs. This can result in angina, heart attack, stroke, kidney failure or the need for amputation of part of the leg.

- There may be narrowing of the blood vessels in the kidney, which can lead to kidney failure.
- Burst or bleeding blood vessels can arise in the eyes and/or there may be swelling of the main nerve in the eye. This can result in sight problems or even blindness.
- Because far more effort than normal is required to push blood through narrowed or hardened arteries, the heart muscles become enlarged. Unfortunately, an increased workload for a prolonged period can result in heart failure.
- Certain kinds of dementia (impaired mental ability) can occur after multiple small strokes.

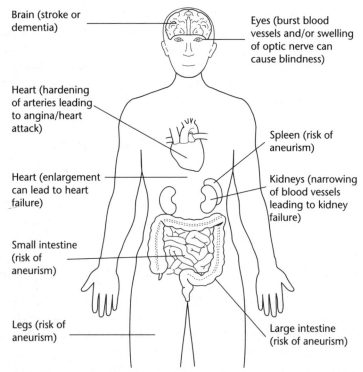

Figure 6 Parts of the body affected by high blood pressure

Angina

Angina is the name given to the severe chest pain that occurs when blood struggles to travel through narrowed arteries in the heart, causing insufficient blood supply to a part or parts of the heart muscle. When you are resting, the blood supply may be enough, but when you are active – maybe walking up the stairs or even just sitting to eat a meal – the extra blood your heart needs to cope with the exertion may not be able to pass the narrowed coronary artery to all areas. The starved area then 'complains' with pain.

Angina is usually treated by a statin drug to lower your cholesterol level – cholesterol deposits are capable of blocking the coronary arteries – as well as low-dose aspirin to prevent a heart attack. In many cases, a beta-blocker drug is also prescribed, as well as another drug in some cases, such as an angiotensin-converting enzyme (ACE) inhibitor (see Chapter 7 for more information on medications). When drugs fail to ease and prevent angina pains, you may be offered surgery to widen or bypass narrowed arteries. Angioplasty is one such procedure and consists of an inflatable balloon being passed by catheter to the diseased site and inflated to enlarge the passage. This is usually a permanent option.

If you think you have angina, you should see your doctor as a matter of urgency.

Further tests

After a diagnosis of high blood pressure, you are likely to be sent for some tests. These may include the following:

- A urine test to check for blood or protein: the presence of either of these things can indicate kidney damage from high blood pressure, even if other kidney function tests are normal (see the next bullet point).
- Blood tests to check kidney function: this involves the measurement of electrolytes, blood urea and creatinine levels. If these blood tests show normal kidney function there can still be some kidney damage, as explained in the bullet point above.
- Special tests (including blood tests, imaging tests and biopsies): these will check adrenal and thyroid gland function.

- A lipid profile (lipids are fats): this measures levels of various kinds of cholesterol.
- An electrocardiogram (known as an ECG) to record your heart rhythm: this is a non-invasive procedure which detects the electrical activity of the heart muscle and records it on paper.
- An echocardiogram: this is an ultrasound examination of the heart taken through the chest in which sound waves transmit images to a video monitor. It can determine the thickness (enlargement) on the main pumping side of the heart (the left side).
- A chest X-ray: this looks inside the heart for possible defects.
- Doppler ultrasound to check blood flow through the arteries at pulse points in the arms, hands, legs and feet: this examination can detect the presence of peripheral vascular disease, which can be linked to high blood pressure. The arteries leading to the kidneys can also be checked in this way.
- An ultrasound scan of the kidneys *or* a CT scan of the abdomen: this will assess kidney and adrenal gland function.
- An eye examination with an opthalmoscope to check for changes in the retina at the back of the eyes: possible eye problems can include small haemorrhages in the retina, narrowing of the small arteries and swelling of the eye nerve.

The above tests should determine whether or not your high blood pressure has been caused by another problem, such as kidney disease or hormonal dysfunction. If a related health problem is found, you will be offered the very latest in treatment and care. With kidney disease and so on, however, there are generally symptoms, meaning that associated high blood pressure is usually found before this point.

The aforementioned tests will also ascertain whether or not your high blood pressure has already affected the size of your heart and its ability to function efficiently. If heart enlargement or other anomalies are detected, you will be given the appropriate treatment.

As raised cholesterol levels and diabetes are frequently found in association with high blood pressure, these conditions are checked for, too. If either or both are found, you will be given the appropriate treatment.

Drug treatment

Your doctor is likely to recommend drug treatment to lower your blood pressure in the following instances:

- if your blood pressure fails to drop below 160/100, despite making any necessary lifestyle changes for a trial period (if your doctor does not mention such a trial period, ask whether he or she agrees that you can try lowering your blood pressure by natural means for a time);
- if your blood pressure fails to drop below 140/90, despite making any necessary lifestyle changes for a trial period, *and* you have diabetes, an existing cardiovascular disease or a strong likelihood of developing cardiovascular disease in the next ten years, as assessed by your doctor;
- if your blood pressure is 130/80 or more and you have had a recent heart attack, stroke, transient ischaemic attack (TIA, usually referred to as a 'mini stroke') or complications from diabetes. You also fall into this category if you have ongoing kidney disease.

Target blood pressure

If you have none of the health problems where good blood pressure control is important (see above), the blood pressure reading you should aim for is 140/90 or below. People with cardiovascular disease, diabetes or chronic kidney disease would be best advised to ask their GP or practice nurse for their target blood pressure.

It is estimated that reducing a high diastolic (the lower figure, or the one to the right) blood pressure by 6 mm Hg reduces the risk of stroke by 35–40 per cent, and the risk of cardiovascular disease by 20–25 per cent. Larger reductions provide even greater benefits.

When to see your doctor

You would be well advised to see your doctor immediately if you experience any of the following symptoms:

- light-headedness or dizziness
- severe headache
- nausea related to the headache
- sudden or gradual changes in vision
- chest pain and/or shortness of breath on exertion.

You need to visit your hospital emergency department urgently if you experience any of the following symptoms:

- feeling faint, combined with severe headache and nausea
- loss of vision (partial or complete)
- chest pain or breathlessness that is either severe or occurs when resting
- unexplained sudden weakness.

If, when your blood pressure is measured by a doctor, it is found to be very high, steps will immediately be taken to lower it.

Low blood pressure

Anyone with a blood pressure reading of 90/60 or lower is classed as having low blood pressure (also referred to as *hypotension*). This is good news for the majority of individuals concerned, as the lower the blood pressure, the less chance there is of heart disease, stroke, and so on, occurring. In a few cases, however, the flow of blood is too low to deliver sufficient oxygen and nutrients to the heart, brain and other vital organs, causing dizziness or fainting in the short term and possible organ damage in the long term. It's important, therefore, that if you experience the above-mentioned symptoms you visit your doctor so that he or she can check for the cause, such as an underlying medical condition or a certain type of medication. Depending upon whether or not an underlying cause is found, your doctor will do one of the following:

- change your medication to one which doesn't affect your blood pressure;

- start treating the underlying medical condition;
- prescribe medication to control your blood pressure.

Defining low blood pressure

Low blood pressure is unlike high blood pressure in that it is defined primarily by signs and symptoms rather than by a specific blood pressure reading. For example, some individuals have a very low reading in the region of 90/50 – but as they are not bothered by dizziness or fainting they don't warrant a diagnosis of low blood pressure. Alternatively, other individuals have a reading in the region of 100/60, but as they do have dizziness and fainting they are likely to be given a diagnosis of low blood pressure.

2

Exercise and being active

Research has shown that people who are physically active have lower average blood pressures and are less likely to develop high blood pressure than those who live a sedentary lifestyle. Indeed, a range of studies have shown that people who are fit are 20 to 50 per cent less likely than their sedentary counterparts to develop high blood pressure at some point. This is because being active and taking regular exercise actually conditions the heart and cardiovascular system so that oxygen can be transported around the body more efficiently. Exercise is therefore a powerful weapon against the condition, particularly when adopted in conjunction with other treatment regimes. Indeed, a healthy diet, stress control, regular exercise and so on can work together to prevent the condition or, in someone who already has high blood pressure, give rise to significant improvement.

If some of your blood pressure readings have been higher than others – yet not high enough for you to have been given a diagnosis of high blood pressure – you can lower your risk of developing 'full-blown' high blood pressure by following a regular exercise regime. It's important to choose the type of exercise you carry out with care, making sure to avoid any activity that may be difficult to keep up, such as swimming at a pool a good distance away. Be flexible, too, as variety keeps exercise interesting and enjoyable. As you read through the exercise possibilities in this chapter, mark the ones you think you can easily do. It's not wise to throw yourself straight into a more challenging routine.

If your doctor recommends that you carry out only gentle exercise, remember that after following the guidelines in this book your blood pressure may drop to a level at which it is safe to expand your routine in time.

Here are some of the benefits of regular exercise:

- It seems to relax the blood vessels.

20

- It decreases stress hormone levels.
- It improves kidney function.
- It aids weight loss in people who are overweight.

Exercise and borderline high blood pressure

Exercise studies have shown that people with blood pressure in the normal to high range who perform moderate intensity cardiovascular exercise for 45 minutes per day at least three times a week have a reduction in blood pressure at rest and during moderate exercise. The types of exercise carried out were brisk walking, jogging, gardening and housework.

If your blood pressure is in the moderate to high range and you are given the 'green light' to exercise by your doctor, pick out the exercises you believe you can easily do.

How quickly does exercise work?

The majority of studies into the effects of exercise on high blood pressure have shown that the body responds quickly. Indeed, resting blood pressure will usually fall within a few weeks, with the most dramatic drop occurring in the very first week. However, when study participants ceased to exercise, their blood pressure rapidly returned to its pre-exercise status. This means that a regular exercise regime is essential for continued benefits.

Exercise and high blood pressure

If you have been diagnosed with high blood pressure it is best to avoid sustained heavy resistance (*isometric exercise*), meaning exercise in which muscle tension is developed without contraction of the muscle. Competitive situations involving strenuous exercise should be avoided, too. Carrying out resistance training solely on its own can, for someone with high blood pressure, cause a sudden drop in blood pressure and consequently fainting. It should therefore never be carried out in isolation and always followed by gradual cool-down exercises, as shown on p. 37.

Blood pressure during exercise

Owing to the increased demand in the muscles for oxygen-rich blood during exercise, it is normal for blood pressure to rise at this time – whether you have high blood pressure or not. What is not normal is for the blood pressure reading in a healthy person to reach very high levels during exercise. This means that, rather than having a normal systolic reading of 160 to 220 while taking vigorous exercise, it may spike at around 250 or higher. An increasing number of experts believe that this may be an early indication of heart disease in individuals whose blood pressure is otherwise normal, and that blood pressure levels should ideally be measured during exercise instead of at rest.

In study participants, it has actually been shown that abnormally high blood pressure during vigorous treadmill exercise is linked to a poorer ability of the blood vessels to expand and allow in more oxygen-rich blood. This appears to occur because, in some people, the *endolithial* cells which line blood vessels fail to dilate sufficiently to handle the extra blood flow. Failure of the endolithial cells to dilate is an indicator of heart disease.

It would perhaps be wise for everyone to have their blood pressure taken while jogging on a treadmill to ascertain whether or not their blood vessels are expanding as expected. However, as impaired endolithial function is associated with ageing, diabetes, the menopause, smoking and high cholesterol levels as well as high blood pressure, the treadmill test is not definitive. It is simply thought to be one of the many risk factors for developing heart disease and it is believed to be too early for researchers to recommend that people have exercise tests just to measure their blood pressure.

Tissue hypoxia and ischaemic heart disease

If you are out of condition for some reason or engaging in an exercise which requires a muscle to use in excess of 25 per cent of its strength, the pressure of blood within the muscle can cause the small blood vessels to collapse. This stops oxygen-rich blood from being pumped into the muscle, giving rise to temporary muscle pain. A lack of oxygen in the muscles is known as *tissue hypoxia*, and creates a rapid increase in blood pressure (both the systolic and diastolic rates) for the duration of muscle contraction. The rise in blood pressure is caused by the small blood vessels being forced open as the body attempts to deliver oxygen to the working muscles.

When blood pressure rises, the strain on the heart quickly increases. This can result in a restriction of the blood flow to the heart muscle in patients who already have heart disease – a condition known as *myocardial ischaemia*, which simply means reduced blood supply to the heart muscle. The main symptom of *stable ischaemic heart disease* (IHD for short) is angina, which is characterized by severe chest pain on exertion and decreased exercise tolerance. The symptoms of *un*stable IHD are chest pain even at rest, or rapidly worsening angina. If you think you may have IHD, speak to your doctor. You should then be referred to your local hospital for either an electrocardiogram, a coronary angiogram, blood tests (to show cardiac markers) or cardiac stress testing. Treatment may include medication, coronary artery bypass surgery or angioplasty – the latter being the insertion of an inflatable balloon into the diseased artery to widen it.

As IHD is believed to be the most common cause of death in most Western countries, don't ever ignore chest pain or worsening angina. If you have high blood pressure, the development of IHD can be prevented by a healthy diet, stress control measures and perhaps medication. Exercise can also be a great preventative measure, but it is important first to get the go-ahead from your doctor.

Don't overdo it

After carrying out warm-up exercises, try to do one or two of the easier stretching exercises. If you have arthritis or another limiting condition which makes your stiffness, fatigue and pain levels higher than normal the following day, either you did not allow sufficient resting time for your body to recover or your chosen exercises were overambitious. Allow your body a further two or three days to recover, then recommence your routine with more basic exercises, and make sure you get enough rest afterwards. As you finish your exercise routine, you should feel as if you could have done more. Bear in mind that you may be able to achieve any dropped exercises when your joints and soft tissues (muscles, ligaments and so on) are stronger.

It is recommended that you think carefully about all the exercises described in this chapter. You may perhaps want to rank the exercises, placing one asterisk against those you think you can attempt, then two asterisks beside the easiest of them, starting your routine with these. You may aim to do 15 minutes' exercise a day, but, to be safe, you should spend only two or three minutes exercising at the outset. On the other hand, your objective may be to exercise for an hour. This is not advisable! It is far safer to break exercise sessions into two parts, completing a second session later in the day if you still feel up to it.

Don't hold your breath!

Many people hold their breath during the contraction phase of the exercise, but doing so during sustained muscle contraction restricts blood flow back to the heart. This reduces the amount of blood available for the heart to pump and perhaps limits the amount of blood flowing to the brain. Therefore, when exercising, you need to always exhale on the exertion (or lifting) phase and inhale on the relaxation (or lowering) phase. Doing this is difficult at first, but quickly becomes easier and more natural.

Can older people exercise?

You may wonder whether older people with high blood pressure can safely exercise. The answer is a resounding 'yes', so long as you check with your doctor first. In studies, older patients with high blood pressure carried out both aerobic exercise and weight training for three hours per week, with no adverse effects on diastolic blood pressure or heart function at the end of the programme. Indeed, for most participants their blood pressure reduced. Other positive effects were an approximate 20 per cent reduction in abdominal fat, together with an average weight loss of 2.2 kg (4 lb).

Regular exercise is also known to have an energizing effect, promotes a reduction in stress, helps to condition the heart muscle and aids in maintaining joint mobility.

Warm-up exercises

Some of your muscle groups may be tight and prone to being painful, particularly if you have arthritis or another limiting condition. If you try to move such muscles beyond a certain point they may resist, and forcing them only makes them more painful. It is essential, therefore, that warm-up exercises are performed at the start of your routine. Warm-ups should include mobility exercises for your joints, simple pulse-raising activities for your heart and lungs and short, static stretches for your muscles.

The warm-up exercises you choose should depend largely on your fitness level and particular limitations. If you are out of condition for some reason, you would be advised to formulate a very gentle programme. One or two repetitions of several exercises are generally better than several repetitions of only one or two exercises. If you are quite fit and have no other health concerns, you should be able to devise a more challenging daily programme, lasting maybe 15 to 30 minutes. Your warm-ups should last up to ten minutes and be slightly more energetic than if you were out of condition.

Note: Never skip warm-ups in favour of more vigorous exercise.

Mobility exercises

Mobility exercises should be smooth and continuous, carried out while your body is in a relaxed state – exercising when tense can cause more harm than good. Remember to keep your back straight, your bottom tucked in and your stomach flattened as you perform your routine. Stand with your legs slightly apart.

Shoulders

Letting your arms hang loose, slowly circle your shoulders backwards. Repeat the exercise two to ten times, depending on your condition. Now slowly circle your shoulders forwards and repeat between two and ten times, as appropriate.

Neck

1 Making sure you are standing straight, slowly turn your head to the left – as far as it will comfortably go – then hold for a count

of two. Return to the centre and repeat the exercise between two and ten times. Now turn your head to the right, holding for a count of two before returning to centre. Repeat between two and ten times.

2 Tucking in your chin, tilt your head down and hold for a count of two. Repeat between two and ten times. Again tucking in your chin, tilt your head upwards, but not so far that it virtually sits on your shoulders, and hold for a count of two. Repeat between two and ten times.

Spine

1 Placing your hands on your hips to help support your lower back, slowly tilt your upper body to the left and hold for a count of two. Return to the centre, then repeat between two and ten times. Now tilt to the right and return to the centre. Repeat between two and ten times (see Figure 7).

2 Keeping your lower back static, gently, in a flowing rather than fast movement, swing your arms and upper body to the left as far as they will comfortably go, then return to the centre. Repeat between two and ten times. Now swing your arms and upper body to the right and return to the centre. Repeat between two and ten times.

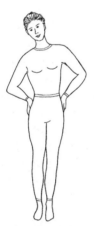

Figure 7 Spine mobility exercise

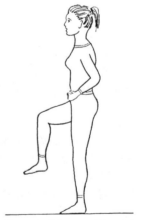

Figure 8 Hips and knees mobility exercise

Hips and knees

With your body upright, move your hips by lifting your left knee upwards, as far as is comfortable. Hold for a count of two, then lower. Now raise your right knee and hold for a count of two before lowering. Repeat between two and ten times (see Figure 8).

Ankles

With your supporting leg slightly bent, place your left heel on the floor in front of you. Lift up your left foot and then place your left toes on the floor. Repeat between two and ten times. Now duplicate the exercise and number of repetitions with the right foot (see Figures 9(a) and (b)).

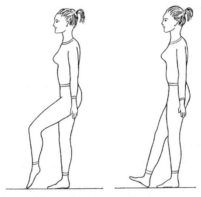

Figures 9(a) and (b) Ankle mobility exercises

Pulse-raising activities

Still part of your warm-up routine, pulse-raising activities must be gentle and should build up gradually. Their purpose is to help warm your muscles in preparation for stretching. Walking around the room for two to four minutes, followed, if possible, by walking once up and down the stairs, is ideal.

Stretching exercises

The muscles, already becoming warm and flexible, relax further when short stretches follow mobility and pulse-raising activities. Stretches prepare them for the more challenging movements that, hopefully, follow. These exercises have been devised with the help of the Health Education Authority.

Again, it is up to you to decide which you think you are capable of performing.

Calves

1 Stand with your arms outstretched, your palms against a wall. Keeping your left foot on the floor, bend your left knee and stretch your right leg out behind you. Press the heel of your right foot into the floor until you feel a gentle stretch in your leg muscles. Now change over legs. Repeat between two and ten times (see Figure 10).

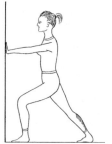

Figure 10 Stretching exercise for the calves

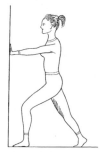

Figure 11 Stretching exercise for the fronts of the thighs

2 Standing with your feet slightly apart, raise both heels off the floor so that you are on your toes. Repeat between two and ten times. As your calf muscles strengthen, you should be able to stay on your toes for longer periods of time. This exercise also helps your balance.

Fronts of the thighs

Using a chair or wall for support, stand with your left leg in front of your right, both knees bent, your right heel off the floor. Tuck in your bottom, and move your hips forwards until you feel a gentle stretch in the front of your right thigh. Now change over legs. Repeat between two and ten times (see Figure 11).

Backs of the thighs

Stand with your legs slightly bent, your left leg about 20 cm (8 in) in front of your right leg. Keeping your back straight, place both hands on your hips and lean forwards a little. Now straighten your left leg, tilting your bottom back, until you feel a gentle stretch in the back of your left thigh. Now change over legs. Repeat between two and ten times (see Figure 12).

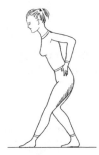

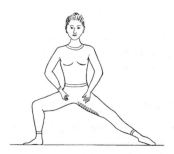

Figure 12 Stretching exercise for the backs of the thighs

Figure 13 Stretching exercise for the inner thigh

Inner thigh

Spreading your legs slightly, your hips facing forwards and your back straight, bend your left leg and, keeping the right leg straight, move it slowly sideways until you feel a gentle stretch along your inner thigh. Gently move to the right, bending your right leg as you straighten the left (see Figure 13).

Chest

Keeping your back straight, your knees slightly bent and your pelvis tucked under, place your arms as far behind your lower back as you can and your hands gently on your lower back. Now move your shoulders and elbows back until you feel a gentle stretch in your chest (see Figure 14 overleaf).

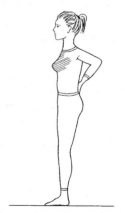

Figure 14 Stretching exercise for the chest

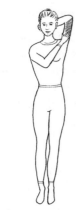

Figure 15 Stretching exercise for the back of the upper arms

Back of the upper arms

With your knees slightly bent, your back straight and your pelvis tucked under, raise your left arm and bend it so that your hand drops behind your neck and upper back. Using your right hand, apply slight pressure backwards and downwards on your left elbow, until you feel a gentle stretch (see Figure 15).

Strengthening exercises

The following exercises help to condition the muscles required for pushing, pulling and lifting. They should also help to increase your stamina. Remember to incorporate small pauses between repetitions, focus on staying relaxed and don't forget to breathe out on each muscle contraction.

Thighs

1 Lean back against a wall, your feet 30 cm (12 in) away from the base of the wall. Adopting correct posture, slowly squat down, keeping your heels on the ground. (Don't go too far down at first.) Now slowly straighten your legs. Repeat between two and ten times, lowering yourself further as, over time, your muscles strengthen.

2 Holding on to a sturdy chair and keeping your back 'tall',
  bend and then slowly straighten both legs, keeping your heels
  on the floor. Repeat the exercise between two and ten times
  (see Figure 16).

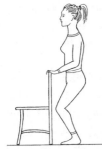

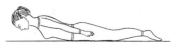

**Figure 17 Strengthening
exercise for the upper back**

**Figure 16 Strengthening
exercise for the thighs**

3 Sit in a chair and push your knees together, tightening your
  thigh muscles as you do so. Hold for a few seconds. Repeat
  between two and ten times.

Upper back

Lie face down on the floor, hands by your side, not on the floor, and
keeping your legs straight and tightening your stomach and back
muscles, gently raise your head and shoulders. Hold for a count of
two, then lower. Repeat between two and ten times (see Figure 17).

Lower back

Lie on your back, using a small rolled cloth or towel to support your
neck if necessary, then lift your knees, keeping your feet on the floor.
Lift first your left leg gently behind the knee, pulling it towards your
chest until you feel a gentle pull in your bottom and lower back.
Repeat with the right leg. Now pull both legs up together. Repeat
each exercise between two and ten times (see Figure 18).

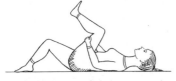

**Figure 18 Strengthening exercise
for the lower back**

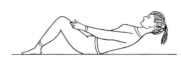

**Figure 19 Strengthening exercise
for the abdomen**

Abdomen

1 Lie on your back, using a small rolled cloth or towel to support your neck if necessary. Lift your knees and place your feet flat on the floor. Now tighten your abdominal muscles, tuck your chin in a little towards your chest and raise your head and shoulders, reaching with your arms towards your knees. Remember to keep your lower back pressed down on the floor (see Figure 19 on the previous page).

2 If you are not fit enough to perform sit-ups, the following exercise is just as effective. Lie on your back, using a small rolled cloth or towel to support your neck if necessary. Pull in your stomach muscles and try to flatten your spine against the floor. Hold for a count of two, then release. Repeat between two and ten times.

Arms

Place your left hand on your chest and press for a few seconds. Do the same with your right arm. Repeat between two and ten times.

Push-ups

Stand with your hands flat against a wall, your body straight. Carefully lower your body towards the wall, then slowly push away. Repeat two to ten times. At first, stand quite near the wall, then try moving further away as you become stronger (see Figures 20(a) and (b)).

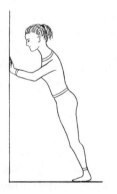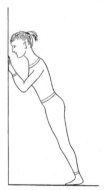

Figures 20(a) and (b) Push-ups

Using small weights

Lifting weights is a great way to increase muscular strength and improve overall physical fitness. You may wish to use the type that fasten with Velcro around your wrists and ankles and are available from most sports shops. Weights of 225 g (8 oz) each slip into small pockets sewn into the band. Start by using one weight only and remember to breathe out as a muscle contracts.

1 With the weights around your wrists, stand with your feet slightly apart. Making sure that only your upper body moves, turn carefully to the left, swinging both arms gently as you move. Repeat two or three times. Now perform the same exercise and number of repetitions, but this time swing your body and arms to the right. Ensure the movements are steady and fluid, not too fast.

2 Keeping your left elbow close to your waist, slowly raise your left forearm so it almost touches your shoulder. Lower the forearm until it is at right angles with your upper arm, then slowly raise it again. Now repeat the exercise with your right arm, again ensuring your movements are steady and continuous.

3 Bending your left arm, bringing your hand up until your wrist is level with your shoulder, reach your hand upwards until your elbow is level with your shoulder. Bring it straight back down to the original position. Repeat once more, then do the same with your right arm.

As you gain in strength and flexibility you may be able, first, to increase the number of repetitions you do and, second, to add to the weight you lift. If you have a chronic pain condition and your pain levels are higher than normal the next day, it is recommended that you postpone these exercises until you feel stronger.

Walking with weights

Strapping the Velcro weight bands around your ankles and placing one weight in each, walk around the house, up and down the stairs or on a treadmill to strengthen your cardiovascular system and the muscles in your legs, hips and back. If you feel only slight discomfort later on, repeat the exercise every day until the discomfort abates. Next, increase the time you spend wearing the weight bands and slowly add more weights.

Aerobic exercise

When we carry out aerobic exercise of some kind, our muscle temperature rises, which helps the muscles to relax. This means they receive more oxygen and waste products are removed more efficiently. Weight training (see p. 33) does not appear to be as effective at lowering blood pressure as aerobic exercise. The cardiovascular system also benefits from aerobic exercise, helping to protect against heart disease, improving circulation and meaning you are less out of breath. Regular aerobic activity also carries the added bonuses of increasing your stamina levels and helping you lose weight.

Ideally, you should aim to develop a programme in which you carry out aerobic exercise three or four times a week, for ten minutes to an hour, starting slowly and building up your time as you feel able.

Note: Check with your doctor before going ahead with *any* aerobic activity.

Walking

Always ensure you choose an aerobic exercise you enjoy and one that is within your physical – and practical – scope. Walking is good. It is a weight-bearing activity that increases mobility, strength and stamina, and helps protect against osteoporosis (thinning bones). If you are very out of condition, you may just want to walk to the nearest lamppost and back on your first day. On the second and third days, you should try to repeat that. On the fourth day, you could try walking to the second lamppost, on the fifth and sixth days to repeat that, on the seventh to the third lamppost, on the ninth and tenth to repeat that and so on. For most people, walking is the easiest and most convenient aerobic activity. You may surprise yourself at how far you actually can walk, after increasing the distance over several weeks.

Unfortunately, walking outdoors is not always practical in the UK climate. An electrically operated treadmill can be an excellent investment giving you the freedom to walk whenever you wish, whatever the weather. Also, as a treadmill offers continuous level walking, people with arthritis or other health problems can walk for far greater distances than they could hope to with the variable terrain outdoors. Some people consider treadmill walking monotonous and artificial, but this can largely be overcome by positioning it near a shelf so you can read a book or magazine at the same time. Another alternative is to listen to your favourite music or podcasts on an MP3 player to help pass the time.

Stepping

If you think 'stepping' is an option for you, start with a small step such as a thick book or maybe a catalogue or telephone directory. Make sure it is placed securely against a bottom stair to keep it steady and give you room to move. After two or three weeks, you may be able to use the bottom stair itself. Place first your left foot, then your right foot on the book or step. Now step backwards with first your left foot, then your right. Repeat between two and ten times, then alternate your feet, placing first your right foot, then your left. If possible, build up your agility until you can do this exercise for about ten minutes.

Trampoline jogging

Jogging on a small, circular trampoline can, if care is taken, provide a great aerobic workout. Get accustomed to the feel of it by first simply lifting your heels – not your feet – as if you are walking. If you can manage to get into a rhythm, the trampoline will do much of the work for you. Continue for two or three minutes per session until you feel able to gradually extend the time to around ten minutes. Small, inexpensive trampolines are available from most sports shops.

Swimming

Swimming is a great exercise with a lower risk of injury than is associated with most other forms of aerobic activity. It has the following benefits:

- It works all the major muscles in the body without causing undue stress on the bones.

- The pressure of the water causes the chest to expand, encouraging deeper breathing and increased oxygen intake.
- It improves blood circulation.
- It doesn't overexert the heart.

If you get tired of swimming laps, try simple kicking, treading water, 'slow' running through the water or jumping on the spot.

If you live near to the swimming baths, try to swim once or twice a week, gradually building up your swimming time to one hour per session. Note that if the baths are a good distance away, you will probably find yourself attending less and less as time goes by until you eventually give up, provoking feelings of failure. You can avoid any such negative feelings by steering clear of activities that are difficult to keep doing on a regular basis.

Aqua-aerobics

Aqua-aerobics (sometimes called 'aqua-cizes') are a pleasing and beneficial form of exercise in the water, particularly if you aren't able to swim. Because the water supports your body as you exercise – when you are submerged to the neck, you bear only about a tenth of your body weight – it removes the shock factor, conditioning your muscles with the minimum of discomfort.

Rather than exercising alone in the baths, most people prefer to join an aqua-aerobics class. As well as providing encouragement and ensuring that you exercise properly for maximum benefit, this can bring you into contact with people who have similar health conditions, such as arthritis, so you can empathize with, and support, each other. Most public swimming baths run aqua-aerobics sessions, some of which are graded according to ability.

Aqua-aerobics, as with all types of exercise, are only truly beneficial when performed regularly.

Cycling

Whether you use an exercise bike or an actual bicycle, this activity provides a good cardiovascular workout. However, caution must rule, especially if you have another health condition such as arthritis, for a small hard seat and handlebars set too far forward can aggravate the problem. Also, owing to the continuous motion, your legs have no opportunity to rest, as they would between spells of most other types of exercise.

Even if you have no additional health concerns, it is still best to start by pedalling slowly, gradually building momentum. Limit your sessions to two or three minutes at first. After a month you may be able to cycle for 20 to 30 minutes.

Cooling-down exercises

Cooling down your muscles after exercise is just as important as warming them up beforehand. You can do this by repeating your choice of warm-up exercises for about five minutes.

Getting started on your routine

So, have you checked with your doctor and made your choices? Have you selected the easier exercises with which you wish to start your routine? If so, you should now read the following recommendations. They should help to get you started with the minimum of discomfort.

First of all, it is advisable to exercise before your pain levels start to rise. It is important, too, that you set aside sufficient time to perform your routine – don't be tempted to rush.

- Relax your muscles by taking a warm shower shortly after waking.
- Eat a light breakfast to boost your energy levels – you should not exercise after a heavy meal.
- Dress in loose, comfortable clothing and good, supportive trainers.
- Ensure that you exercise in a warm place, out of draughts.
- Start slowly and carefully. Be sure to perform only two or three repetitions of your chosen exercises.
- Movements should be kept within your range. If you know that raising your arms past a certain level gives rise to pain in your shoulder, make sure you don't initially pass that level. You should actually be able to extend your range with time.
- As you exercise, keep checking your posture. When you allow

your head and shoulders to droop, your back to slouch, you put added strain on your muscles. They then burn more energy, causing additional pain and fatigue.

- Take care that you don't involuntarily hold your breath when exercising. Breathe deeply and evenly, breathing out on the effort.
- Try to visualize the muscle group being exercised. This should prevent other muscle groups accidentally being worked.
- Ensure you pause between repetitions. As there is a slight delay between muscle contraction and relaxation, contracting a muscle without pausing means you do so when the muscle has already contracted. This causes a build-up of lactic acid in the area concerned, which, in turn, causes pain.
- After exercising, it is important to allow time for recovery before attempting further activity. Don't berate yourself if your pain levels are surprisingly high afterwards. Get some extra rest, then begin a toned-down version of your routine as soon as you are able.
- When you finish you should feel as if you could have done more. This should ensure you don't set yourself up for more pain for later.
- Don't try to make up for the days when you weren't able to do much. Set your limit at the start of each session and stick to it.

Tips for being more active

You can add more physical activity into your daily routine in the following ways:

- Ride a bike instead of travelling by car.
- If you must use a car, park further away from your place of work.
- If you take the bus, get off one or two stops early and walk the remaining distance.
- Use the stairs instead of the lift.
- Clean the house regularly.
- Instead of using a drive-in carwash, clean the car by hand.
- Take up gardening.
- Take up dancing.

3

Food and nutrition

What a person eats and drinks has a definite effect on heart and blood pressure, as well as overall health. A junk food diet, for example, containing a lot of sugar and salt, chemical additives and refined carbohydrates (such as cakes, pastries, biscuits, sweets, sweetened fruit juice, etc.), and so on, is treated as toxic by the body and can result in chronic illness. A balanced wholefood diet, on the other hand, can only promote good health. It can also prevent unwanted weight gain and help you to achieve the optimum weight for your size.

A balanced wholefood diet

Wholefoods are simply those that have had nothing taken away – i.e. nutrients and fibre – and that have had nothing added – i.e. colourings, flavourings and preservatives. In short, they are foods in their most natural form (see Figure 21). Wholefoods that

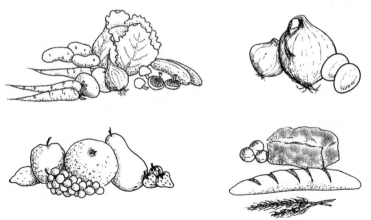

Figure 21 Foods to eat

are organically produced – without the use of potentially dangerous chemical fertilizers, pesticides and herbicides – are even better for us.

Fresh fruit and vegetables

Studies have shown that eating more fruit and vegetables can help to lower blood pressure. Fruit and vegetables are rich in vitamins, minerals, fibre and enzymes which work together to keep your body in good condition. However, vitamin C is quickly used up in the body by smoking, alcohol consumption, surgery, trauma, stress, exposure to pollutants and the use of certain medications.

Fruit such as bananas, prunes, cantaloupe and honeydew melon and dried peaches and apricots are high in potassium, too, which is important for counteracting the negative effects of salt. In effect, lowering salt levels within the body can directly lower blood pressure. Bananas are extremely high in potassium yet low in salt, which makes eating a couple of them daily a great way to help lower high blood pressure.

Eating onions, celery and garlic on a daily basis has been shown in studies to reduce systolic blood pressure in people with high blood pressure. It is best to consume about 4 g of fresh garlic per day. If you don't like eating garlic, try taking a high-potency garlic pearl or capsule. Should this repeat on you, try keeping them in the fridge and taking while very cold – they will then melt further down in your stomach.

Select locally grown, organic fruit and vegetables that are in season – these have the highest nutrient content and the greatest enzyme activity. Organically grown products may not look as perfect as those that are processed, but they *are* superior. Try to eat as fresh and as raw as possible. When you have to cook your vegetables, use unsalted (or lightly salted) water and simmer for the minimum length of time. Lightly steaming and stir-frying are healthy alternatives. Scrub rather than peel your vegetables.

Some other eating suggestions are listed below:

- Eat a range of different fruits to add more interest. Different fruits provide different nutrients.

- If you work, pack an orange, banana or grapes to snack on during the day.
- Dried apricots, peaches and pineapple slices store well so you can keep a bag of them in your drawer at work to snack on.
- Add crushed fresh pineapple to coleslaw and cottage cheese and add mandarin oranges or grapes to a tossed salad.
- Have baked apples, pears or a fruit salad for dessert.
- When buying tinned fruit, choose fruit soaked in 100 per cent fruit juice rather than in syrup.
- Make a variety of green salads and try to eat one every day.
- Varying your vegetables will make your meals more interesting. Also, a wide variety ensures that your body gets all the nutrients it needs.
- Buy packets of baby carrots or celery sticks to snack on.
- To make a quick meal when you aren't feeling too good, it's okay to buy tinned vegetables. Look for labels saying 'no salt added'. If you feel you then need to add a small pinch of salt yourself, it will still amount to far less than that in a normal tin of vegetables.
- Plan some meals around vegetables rather than around meat. Examples are vegetable stir-fry, vegetable curry and vegetable soup.
- Add chopped vegetables to a pasta sauce or lasagne.
- To thicken and flavour a soup, stew or gravy, use cooked and pureed vegetables such as potatoes.
- When preparing a barbecue meal, try grilled vegetable kebabs.
- Don't buy vegetables that come with sauces. They are likely to contain a lot of added salt, sugar or fats.
- Frozen, dried and tinned vegetables are as good as fresh, provided they don't contain added salt and sugar.
- Eat fresh fruit and vegetables as soon as possible to avoid nutrient loss. If you don't wish to eat them straight away, freeze them.
- Don't soak prepared fruit or vegetables as the vitamins and minerals can dissolve away.

You will have heard that we should all eat five portions of fruit and vegetables a day, but may not know how to measure a portion. Well, one portion weighs about 80 g (just under 3 oz) and is roughly the size of your fist.

The following amounts illustrate a portion:

- one medium-sized fruit (banana, apple, pear, orange)
- one slice of a large fruit (melon, pineapple, mango)
- two smaller fruits (plums, satsumas, apricots, peaches)
- a dessert bowl full of salad
- three heaped tablespoonfuls of vegetables
- three heaped tablespoons of pulses (chickpeas, lentils, beans)
- two or three tablespoons of grapes or berries
- one tablespoon of dried fruit
- one glass (150 ml or 5 fl oz) of unsweetened fruit or vegetable juice. (If you drink two or more glasses of juice, it still only counts as one portion.)

Legumes (peas and beans)

Legumes are very cheap to buy and contain high amounts of protein, which is vital to the body for growth and maintenance. Protein is directly responsible for approximately 20 per cent of the material in our tissues and cells, and it functions as hormones, antibodies and enzymes – all of which keep the body functioning smoothly.

The soya bean is a complete protein, of which there are many derivatives including soya milk, tofu, tempeh and miso. Tofu, for example, is very versatile and can be used in both savoury and sweet dishes. Soya milk can be used as an alternative to cow's milk.

Seeds

Sunflower, sesame, hemp, flax and pumpkin seeds are very important for strengthening the immune system. They can be eaten as they are as a snack, sprinkled on to salads and cereals, or used in baking. For more flavour they can be lightly roasted and coated with organic soy sauce. Cracked linseed and pumpkin seeds are also highly nutritious and useful for treating constipation. They can be used in baking and sprinkled on to breakfast cereals, over salads, soups and porridge oats.

Nuts

Nuts, too, are an intrinsic part of strengthening the immune system. All nuts contain vital nutrients, but almonds, cashews, walnuts, Brazils and pecans perhaps offer the greatest array. Eat a wide assortment as snacks, with cereal and in baking. Obviously, if you are allergic to nuts, they must be avoided at all costs.

Fibre

Fibre, in the form of wholegrain foods and wholemeal flours, is rich in complex unrefined carbohydrates, which are excellent for health. It also works in synergy with other essential nutrients like calcium, potassium and magnesium, allowing blood pressure to be more easily controlled, particularly if you can take other steps to lower it (as described in this book).

Consuming at least three servings of wholegrain foods daily will not only help to prevent high blood pressure and its associated diseases, it can also help you to achieve your optimum weight – being overweight is one of the risk factors for developing high blood pressure. Indeed, studies have shown that, for each daily serving of wholegrains, a person's chance of getting high blood pressure is likely to fall by about 4 per cent. Other studies have shown that people consuming four servings a day are as much as 23 per cent less likely to develop the condition. When you also take other steps to lower your blood pressure, the estimated drop in your risk is even greater.

With the exception of wheat, aim to consume a variety of grains, including oats, rye, barley (generally available as pearl barley), corn, buckwheat, brown rice and mixed grains. Brown rice, millet, buckwheat and maize or corn are all gluten-free and invaluable to people with a gluten allergy or sensitivity.

Here are some further tips for eating wholegrains:

- Try to eat a bowl of porridge for breakfast every day, buy oatmeal biscuits and oat cereal bars.
- Use brown rice instead of white.
- If you can eat wheat, use wholewheat pasta instead of refined white pasta.
- Use wholegrains such as barley in soups and stews.

- Use bulgur wheat in casseroles and stir-fries.
- Make a pilaf with wholegrains such as wild rice, brown rice and barley.
- Substitute half the refined white flour in pancakes, buns and other flour-based recipes for wholewheat or oat flour.
- Use rolled oats or crushed unsweetened wholegrain cereal to 'bread' chicken, fish, veal cutlets and so on.
- Use wholegrain flour or oatmeal when making baked treats.
- As the colour of a grain is not an indication of whether it is 'whole' or not, read the ingredient list.

Fats and oils

Fats (fatty acids) are the most concentrated sources of energy in our diet, 1 g of fat providing the body with nine calories of energy. They are also a fine source of essential fatty acids (EFAs) which improve circulation and oxygen uptake. Our bodies are unable to manufacture EFAs so they can only come from our diets. A deficiency in EFAs is linked with muscle-tissue wasting, reduced immune-system function and diminished cognitive ability.

There are two distinct types of fatty acids – one bad, one good:

- *Saturated fat* Believed to be implicated in the development of heart disease, saturated fat comes mainly from animal sources and is generally solid at room temperature. Although margarine was, for many years, believed to be a healthier choice over butter, nutritionists have now revised their opinion, for some of the fats in the margarine hydrogenation process are changed into trans-fatty acids which the body metabolizes as if they were saturated fatty acids – the same as butter. Butter is a valuable source of oils and vitamin A, but should be used very sparingly. Margarine, on the other hand, is an artificial product containing many additives, which are not recommended.
- *Unsaturated fat* Also called polyunsaturated or monounsaturated fat, unsaturated fat has a protective effect on the heart and other organs. Omega 3 and omega 6 oils occur naturally in oily fish (mackerel, herring, sardines, tuna, etc.), nuts and seeds, and is usually liquid at room temperature. It is recommended, then, that you eat oily fish at least three times a week and cold-pressed

oil (olive, rapeseed, safflower and sunflower oil) daily, for dressings and in cooking.

It is possible to cut out saturated fats by reading the food label. This should say whether the food in question is 'low fat', 'low in saturated fat', 'medium fat', 'medium in saturated fat', 'high fat' or 'high in saturated fat'. These translate to the following:

- Low means less than 3 g total fat or 1 g saturated fat per 100 g of food. 'Low fat' or 'low in saturated fat' is a good choice.
- Medium means between 3 g and 20 g total fat or 1–5 g saturated fat per 100 g of food. It is recommended that you eat only small amounts of 'medium fat' or 'medium in saturated fat', on an occasional basis.
- High means more than 20 g total fat or 5 g saturated fat per 100 g of food. High fat products should be avoided altogether.

Eggs

Contrary to long-held opinion, the cholesterol in eggs is not now thought to be a risk factor in arterial disease. Indeed, research has shown that egg cholesterol has a clinically insignificant effect on levels of blood cholesterol. Eggs also contain lecithin, a superb biological detergent capable of breaking down fats so they can be utilized by the body. In addition, lecithin prevents the accumulation of too many acid or alkaline substances in the blood and encourages the transport of nutrients through the cell walls. Buy free-range eggs and eat them soft-boiled or poached, as a hard yolk will bind the lecithin, rendering it useless as a fat-detergent.

The Food Standards Agency now states that most people don't need to limit their consumption of eggs so long as they are part of a balanced diet.

Red meat

As red meat is often loaded with saturated fat, it should be eaten in moderation. Look for organically produced meat as the pesticides, antibiotics and hormones used in animal husbandry are an ongoing health issue. If you can't bear to go without red meat, make your serving no larger or thicker than the palm of your hand, and don't eat red meat more than three times a week.

Unfortunately, reducing your consumption of red meat will lower your protein intake. You should therefore ensure that you eat plenty other protein-containing foods such as fish, poultry, soya products, cottage cheese, organic live yogurt, nuts, seeds and legumes. Low protein intake causes the body to pull protein from the muscles, causing weakness, low energy, low stamina, poor resistance to infection and depression.

Here are some suggestions for buying, cooking and eating red meat:

- Choose the leanest cuts of meat you can find. The leanest beef cuts include top loin, top sirloin and shoulder. The leanest pork cuts include pork loin, tenderloin and ham. The leanest lamb cuts are from the shank half of the leg.
- Trim away any visible fat before cooking.
- Grill, roast, poach or boil red meat instead of frying.
- If you must fry your meat on the odd occasion, don't bread it as this adds fat and causes the meat to soak up more fat.
- Choose extra-lean minced meat.
- Any fat that arises from cooking should be carefully drained off.
- Hams, sausages, frankfurters, burgers and luncheon meats are processed and contain added sodium (salt). Unless it says 'low sodium content' on the label, they should be avoided.
- As lower-fat processed meats are now available in shops, check out the nutrition facts on the label and choose processed meats with less saturated fat.

Fish

Fish is a nutritious alternative to red meat. It is particularly beneficial as it is an excellent source of omega 3 fatty acids, gamma linoleic acid (GLA) and the amino acids our bodies need to build protein. Choose coldwater fish, especially oily fish such as sardines, fresh tuna, anchovies, mackerel, trout, salmon, herring (kippers) and pilchards.

- Avoid frying fish. Poach, grill or bake instead.
- Avoid covering fish in breadcrumbs as this adds more fat and makes the fish soak up additional fat.

Poultry

Poultry such as chicken and turkey contains far less fat than red meat, and is a good source of protein and essential fatty acids (EFAs), which can improve blood circulation and oxygen uptake. It is therefore recommended that you eat chicken or turkey once or twice a week.

- The leanest poultry choices are boneless chicken breasts and turkey cutlets.
- Fresh chicken and turkey is usually 'flavour enhanced' by the addition of sodium (salt).
- Avoid poultry with 'self-basting' on the label as this is an indication of sodium addition.
- Even better, look for 'organic' and 'free range' on the label.

Foods to avoid

Reducing or eliminating your intake of the foods mentioned in this section can help to reduce your blood pressure and keep it down (see Figure 22). In some people it will make a dramatic difference and remove the necessity for taking prescription drugs for high blood pressure.

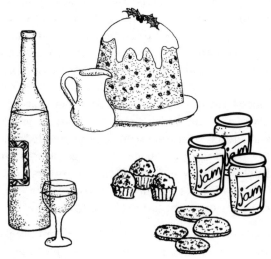

Figure 22 Foods to avoid

Salt

An excess of salt (sodium chloride) is always of great detriment to the body as it forces it to retain too much fluid. This higher volume of fluid throughout the body is the characteristic that can, in a susceptible person, give rise to high blood pressure or worsen existing high blood pressure. High fluid levels circulating through the brain can mean that any weaknesses in the brain's vascular system are revealed, perhaps even resulting in a burst blood vessel – the precursor of a stroke or the cause of blindness in one eye. With intake of too much salt, there is also a greater volume of fluid passing through the heart, which puts it under enormous strain and increases the chances of heart disease.

Note that if you take blood pressure medication and continue to eat a lot of salt there is a good chance that the medication will not be as effective as it could be. This applies to people on blood pressure medication who continue to drink excess alcohol, smoke, avoid exercise, eat a poor diet and/or are prone to stress.

So how much salt is too much? According to a government recommendation, adults should not eat in excess of 6 g of salt a day – however, most people consume 6–10 g daily. Experts believe that if we all cut down our salt intake to no more than 6 g a day, as many as 70,000 heart attacks and strokes a year in the UK would be prevented. It's a real shame that high levels of salt are added as a preservative and flavour-enhancer to most processed and pre-packaged foods and that sodium is present in the commonly used flavouring monosodium glutamate (known as MSG), as well as sodium bicarbonate. For example, just one 400 g tin of soup contains more than 6 g of salt! It's also a fact that surprisingly large amounts of salt are added to such things as bread, biscuits and breakfast cereals, with the exception of shredded wheat products.

Eighty per cent of the salt the average person consumes comes from processed foods and only 20 per cent comes from that used in cooking and added at the table. It is recommended, therefore, that you limit your intake of salt in the following ways:

- Reduce your consumption of processed and pre-packaged foods.
- When you must buy processed and pre-packaged foods, look for 'low salt' or 'sodium-free' on the label. 'Low salt' contains 0.25 g

of salt per 100 g of food, 'medium salt' contains 0.25–1.25 g per 100 g and 'high salt' contains 1.25 g or more of salt.

- If the label doesn't state the amount of salt in a particular food, look at the list of ingredients. The closer salt is to the top of the list, the more salt is contained in the food.
- Use only a very small amount of sea salt or rock salt in baking and cooking.
- Try to avoid sprinkling any type of salt over your meals. People often use salt out of habit.
- Herbs and spices can provide extra flavour, as can seasonings. Examples are ginger, lime juice, lemon juice, garlic and chilli.
- Ketchup, pickled items, mustard, yeast extract and stock cubes, and so on, can contain high levels of salt. Check the label as there are often low-salt alternatives.
- Smoked meat and fish are high in salt. If possible, avoid them.
- If you love a salty flavour to your foods, try using a small sprinkling of a low-sodium salt substitute.
- Use a low-salt cookbook or surf the internet for low-salt recipes.
- If the food label gives the sodium content instead of the salt content, multiply the figure by two and a half to find out the salt content.

You'll be relieved to know that it's not actually necessary to be aware of the exact amount of salt you eat. Simply trying always to eat pre-packaged foods with the lowest salt content and sticking closely to the advice above should make a great difference. Your meals are likely to taste fairly bland at first, but taste buds adjust very quickly to new flavours. Indeed, in the space of a few weeks you will probably wonder why you used to prefer your foods so salty.

Sugar

Sugar consumption has been linked with many disorders, from diabetes to heart disease and cancer. We do need a certain amount of sugar in our diets for conversion to energy, but that can be obtained naturally from foods such as fruits and complex carbohydrates.

If you really must sweeten your food and drinks, alternatives to refined white sugar include raw honey and barley malt. Muscovado and demerara (both of which are often referred to as 'soft brown sugar') are formed during the early stages of the sugar refining process and so contain more nutrients than refined white sugar. They can be used in cooking and baking.

It is not advisable to replace refined white sugar with a sugar substitute such as aspartame, which is sold under the brand names of NutraSweet, Spoonful, Equal and Indulge. Aspartame is an excitatory neurotransmitter (nerve transmitter) that causes nerve cells to fire continually until they become exhausted – and of course this is detrimental to our health.

Many people consume food and drinks containing aspartame in an attempt to lose weight. You may be surprised to learn, though, that this artificial sweetener creates a craving for simple carbohydrates such as cakes, pastries, biscuits and so on, which only gives rise to an increase in weight. When the person stops using aspartame – in diet drinks, for example – he or she generally loses weight. Fortunately, there are natural sweeteners such as Stevia and Xylitol that are perfectly safe and available from health food shops.

Caffeine

Caffeine products – which include coffee, tea, cocoa, cola drinks, energy drinks and chocolate – are stimulants, meaning they make you feel more awake and alert. Caffeine does this by distinctly increasing blood flow, a side effect of which can be blood vessel constriction. Studies have shown that the resulting rise in blood pressure is very short-lived and as yet there is no evidence to link caffeine intake with high blood pressure. I would imagine, however, that people who drink and eat caffeine products many times throughout the day can cause their blood pressure to be almost permanently raised.

Caffeine products can also lead to exhaustion of the adrenal glands, as a result of which the body finds it difficult to cope with stress – and stress is one of the exacerbating factors in high blood pressure. In addition, caffeine products are toxic to the liver, are detrimental to the nervous system and can reduce the body's ability to absorb vitamins and minerals. My best advice is to remove caffeine products from your diet. Fortunately, caffeine is quickly 'washed out' of the system – and it is possible to minimize withdrawal symptoms by reducing your intake over several weeks.

A problem for many is finding an acceptable alternative. Coffee, tea, cocoa and cola drinks can be replaced by fruit juices, vegetable juices and herbal teas (green tea is very good, as is rooibos (redbush) tea) – both are low in tannin and high in beneficial antioxidants. A variety of grain coffee substitutes may also be purchased from health food shops. Because many decaffeinated products are processed with the use of chemicals, they are not a good choice.

Alcohol

Alcohol is a socially acceptable drug, often part of celebrations, casual get-togethers and daily working life. It works as a relaxant, releasing inhibitions and ensuring a good time in the company of others. Alcohol also makes the mind less able to reason, in some cases with aggression as the end result. It is also a depressant, slowing down the reactions and the way the body functions. There are a lot of calories in alcohol, too, and when drunk on a regular basis it makes you put on weight – which will lead to high blood pressure in a susceptible person.

When alcohol is drunk a lot socially, the individual concerned can be surprised at how much he or she actually consumes in a week. However, it's people who wish to block out emotional pain or who have low self-esteem who are more likely than others to drink to excess. Alcohol abuse is a huge problem in the Western world, with one in four adults frequently drinking quantities that can be dangerous to their health.

For women, the maximum safe daily intake is no more than two to three units, with some alcohol-free days in between. For men it is three to four units with some alcohol-free days in between. The weekly safe limit for women is no more than 14 units, and for men it is a maximum of 21 units.

So what is a unit?

- Half a pint of normal strength beer, lager or cider equals one unit.
- One small (100 ml) glass of wine equals one unit.
- A large (175 ml) glass of wine equals two units.
- A single (25 ml) measure of spirits equals one unit.

- One 275 ml bottle of alcopop (5.5 per cent/volume) equals 1.5 units.

It is generally accepted that for a woman to drink more than 35 units of alcohol a week is dangerous to her health. For a man, the danger level is 50 units. If you already have high blood pressure, continuing to drink a lot of alcohol will make your blood pressure rise even more. It will therefore greatly increase your chances of serious health consequences arising. Liver damage is another common outcome of excess alcohol intake, as is damage to other organs and systems in the body.

So how much drink does it take for you to be an alcoholic? A practical definition of alcoholism is persistent drinking that interferes with your health, legal position, interpersonal relationships or means of livelihood. In the UK, there are 4,000,000 heavy drinkers, 800,000 problem drinkers and 400,000 dependent drinkers, or alcoholics.

Your answers to these questions may help you to decide whether or not you are addicted to alcohol:

- Do you regularly drink more than you intended?
- Do you crave drink for much of the time?
- Do you drink to escape worries or troubles?
- Do you feel guilty about your drinking?
- Is your drinking causing a problem in any area of your life – for example, relationships, work, finances, legal or health?
- Does anyone frequently complain about your drinking?

If you have answered 'yes' to two or more of these questions, I'm afraid you have a serious problem. To check on your health situation, it is advisable that you request a medical examination, including a blood pressure check. People in the early stages of alcohol addiction are likely to have not yet developed serious problems.

Starting to accept that alcohol is a problem in your life has to be your first important step towards recovery. If you have tried and failed to overcome your addiction in the past, give yourself another chance. You don't have to tackle the problem alone – there are several responsible organizations which help people to defeat their alcoholism, the main one being Alcoholics Anonymous (see the 'Useful addresses' section on p. 113 for details).

A good diet helps you to maintain a healthy weight

We all store excess energy in our fat cells for our bodies to draw on in times of need – i.e. such as when we eat too little through illness or during a shortage of available food. Eating a healthy balanced diet (such as that discussed in this chapter) will normally ensure that our fat cells store enough energy in reserve but are not over-loaded. It also helps us to maintain a healthy weight. However, it's becoming increasingly common for people in Western societies to eat to excess – and what they do eat is likely to come under the 'junk food' label. As a result, their fat cells store far more energy than they need and they become obese.

Obesity

Obesity in itself is considered a medical condition. This is because of the following:

- Obese people are at increased risk of developing high blood pressure.
- The arteries and other blood vessels can become blocked by cholesterol deposits.
- Obese people are more likely to get other diseases such as diabetes, heart disease, stroke, arthritis and some kinds of cancer.
- Excess weight can exert a lot of strain on the bones and joints.

Blood pressure is more easily controlled in people who are not carrying extra weight. Indeed, studies suggest that approximately 70 per cent of obese adults have high blood pressure. This means that the heart must pump harder than normal to ensure the blood supply reaches all parts. The heavier a person's body weight is, the higher his or her blood pressure is likely to be. Also, people who carry their weight around their waists (known as 'apple-shapes') are more likely than 'pear-shapes' (who carry their weight around their hips and thighs) to have high blood pressure.

Medical professionals have developed a scale which tells you how much excess weight you are carrying. This measure – called the body mass index (BMI) – takes your height into account (see Figure 23). Your doctor will be able to inform you of your current BMI and your optimum BMI. Ideally, we should all have a BMI of not more than 15 per cent above our optimum BMI.

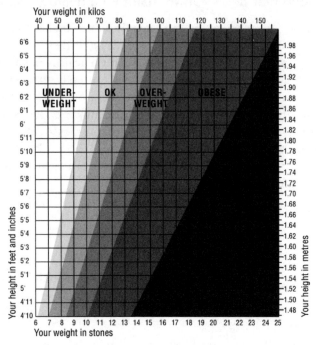

Figure 23 Height–weight chart

If you are overweight

Research has shown that being overweight more than doubles a person's chances of developing high blood pressure. About 70 per cent of overweight adults already have high blood pressure and the height of a blood pressure reading generally corresponds with the degree of obesity. Indeed, a blood pressure reading is likely to increase for every kilogram an overweight person puts on.

You may wonder whether it's possible for a very overweight person to lower his or her blood pressure by making positive life-style changes but not losing weight. The simple answer is that this is unlikely. Changing to healthy eating will, however, effectively bring about weight loss – and without the need for you to half-starve yourself. As even a small amount of weight loss can bring down your blood pressure, you will soon see changes in your blood pressure readings until eventually they are within the normal range.

Changing to healthy eating means getting into the habit of eating healthy foods for the rest of your life. Don't even think about crash dieting or trying to follow a 'fad' diet such as the cabbage soup diet – they are impossible to maintain on a lifelong basis and can be dangerous, too.

If you have changed to a healthy eating diet yet find that you are not losing weight, you should ensure you have smaller helpings of high calorie foods such as meat and cheeses and avoid returning for seconds. You may also need to increase your physical activity to burn up more calories. It may be wise to write down what you eat and when you eat it, too, as you may be automatically snacking on high calorie foods like crisps and chocolate instead of fresh fruits, cereal bars, dried fruit and nuts, etc.

Other useful foods and supplements

- *Ginger* This spice has been found to lower blood pressure in a safe and effective manner. It is therefore one of the most active ingredients you can add to your daily diet. Ginger has a strong, spicy taste that will most probably eliminate any craving for salt. It is commonly used as a seasoning for soups, salads, meats, poultry and many Asian dishes.
- *Omega 3 oils* In studies, omega 3 oils have been shown to help reduce high blood pressure by up to 9 mm Hg. It is best to limit your intake of animal fats and increase your intake of omega 3 oils in the form of cold-pressed vegetable oils – taking approximately 1 tbsp daily is best. Use the oil for making salad dressings and mixing into mashed potatoes and soups. Omega 3 oils are also present in oily fish and should be eaten three times a week. If you find this difficult to do, try taking a good-quality fish oil supplement (not cod-liver oil) and/or a flaxseed oil supplement.
- *Vitamin E* This remarkably safe vitamin has many benefits for the cardiovascular system. It has an oxygen-sparing effect on heart muscle, it aids in the strengthening and regulation of the heartbeat, it helps to break down blood clots and prevent more from forming, and it encourages improved circulation in the smaller

blood vessels. When used to help treat heart attacks, angina, acute and chronic heart disease and high blood pressure, it has been seen to work very well. Doctors have found that it is safe to use quantities as high as 3200 IU daily, which is many times more than the recommended daily dosage. Follow the label instructions very carefully and ensure that you are not buying a synthetic vitamin.

- *Vitamin C* This very safe vitamin has been found to be comparable with prescription medications in lowering high blood pressure. This is because it protects levels of nitrous oxide in the body, which is vital to blood vessel function. Indeed, nitrous oxide relaxes blood vessels and helps to normalize blood pressure. Researchers have found that a 500 mg supplement of vitamin C daily can significantly reduce high blood pressure.

- *B-complex vitamins* The eight vitamins that make up the 'B' group are vitamin B1 (thiamine), vitamin B2 (riboflavin), vitamin B3 (niacin), vitamin B6 (pyridoxine), vitamin B12 (cobalamine), folic acid, pantothenic acid and biotin. Together, these vitamins are very effective at aiding relaxation and lowering stress and anxiety levels. As stress and high blood pressure are closely related, it's advisable to take a B-complex supplement daily. Follow the label dosage instructions.

- *Magnesium* Over 300 biochemical processes are dependent upon this naturally occurring mineral, making it essential for the proper functioning of the body. Initial studies have found that magnesium has a protective effect on the cardiovascular system and plays an important part in regulating blood pressure. People who eat a magnesium-rich diet do seem to be less likely to develop high blood pressure, but there is not enough research as yet to be sure. As this mineral cannot harm, it's recommended that you take it. Follow the label instructions very carefully.

4

Smoking

Although raised activity levels and a healthy diet are important factors in lowering blood pressure (and keeping it down), there are several more lifestyle changes you can make to ensure the optimum outcome. If you smoke, giving it up is a major step in lowering your blood pressure and your risk of developing a variety of serious health problems. This chapter aims to inform you about the many health risks of smoking and takes you step by step through a quitting programme.

If you don't smoke or have already quit, that's really great. You already stand a better chance of avoiding heart disease and the other problems related to high blood pressure. Please skip this chapter.

This chapter refers to any use of tobacco products.

The addictiveness of smoking

The vast majority of smokers are aware that the habit of smoking is harmful, yet many fail to find the willpower required to quit. This state of affairs comes about largely because the nicotine in cigarettes is highly addictive. A person who starts smoking becomes addicted very quickly to the nicotine they contain, developing an irresistible dependence to the extent that stopping would create severe physical and emotional disturbance, known collectively as 'withdrawal symptoms'. Withdrawal symptoms occur because the body is attempting to readjust to functioning without nicotine. Of course, the thought of experiencing withdrawal symptoms is hardly conducive to quitting.

Emotional effects

When smoke is inhaled, nicotine enters the bloodstream through the lungs and the lining of the mouth. The immediate emotional effects are as follows:

- It has a calming effect, especially when delivered to the body in times of stress.
- It activates the 'pleasure centres' in the brain, causing the smoker to experience a 'buzz', or a temporary feeling of euphoria.

The calming effect of nicotine and the sensation of pleasure it brings are clearly enjoyable and rewarding. They are what makes smoking addictive. Add to that the knowledge that attempting to quit will cause emotional anguish and physical problems – even though on a temporary basis – and it's no wonder that smokers find it very tough to give up. Indeed, smokers are often vehement that they don't want to give up the habit and strongly resist any encouragement to do so from the people who care about them.

Physical effects

Smoking also causes physical addiction, producing the following reactions in the body:

- The nicotine in cigarettes acts adversely on some of the brain's chemical messengers (called neurotransmitters), whose function is to send messages from nerve to nerve. Nicotine actually operates as if it was acetylcholine – one of the chief neurotransmitters within the nervous system. As a result, many physiological functions of the brain systems are altered.
- Repeated nicotine intake causes the body to believe that too much acetylcholine is being produced. It responds to this by growing extra acetylcholine receptors.

It can be seen that repeated delivery of nicotine causes structural and functional changes in the brain. Sudden withdrawal of nicotine, then, creates disturbances in the brain and other parts of the body as it attempts to adjust to functioning without nicotine. These disturbances are the body trying to normalize itself and are known collectively as 'withdrawal syndrome'.

Social and psychological effects

There are numerous social and psychological triggers that stimulate the addictive urge to smoke:

- Smoking is like all drug addictions in that the individual quickly learns which circumstances allow him or her to get the maximum rewards from the drug. In other words, people discover when, where and how to take the drug so they most enjoy (in the case of smoking) its smell, taste and handling. For example, a particular person may quickly identify that smoking is enjoyable when taking a coffee break, after a meal and talking on the phone.
- Anxiety, anger and other negative emotions are triggers that bring on the urge to smoke.

Other reasons that smoking is addictive

The modern cigarette is very efficient at rapidly delivering nicotine to the brain. This is because the smoke is 'mild' and so can be inhaled deeply into the lungs. The lungs have a large surface area which allows nicotine to be rapidly absorbed into the bloodstream, reaching the brain within seven seconds.

The quick delivery to the brain is like a small injection of nicotine after each puff. A person who smokes 20 cigarettes a day, each puffed ten times, is self-administering over 70,000 'injections' a year. With each experience of euphoria, the individual becomes more addicted. Cigarettes make smokers feel good and it's only natural to want to feel that way again and again. Of course, some people are satisfied on less nicotine than others.

Smokers take in between 0.5 mg and 2 mg of nicotine from each cigarette, depending upon their preferred needs. They unconsciously regulate their intake by adjusting their puff size, rate of puffing and amount of inhalation, maintaining roughly the same intake from day to day. Two mg of nicotine can be obtained from the same type of cigarette from which another person obtains only 0.5 mg.

How smoking affects the body

It's a fact that smokers risk losing their lives to a cruel disease in exchange for the pleasure of smoking. Indeed, smoking causes many premature deaths from diseases that would not have arisen if the person had managed to quit. It also causes the early onset of a disease that was 'pre-programmed' to happen anyway.

- The main killing diseases related to smoking are heart disease, stroke, vascular disease, cancer and lung problems such as emphysema (the abnormal dilation of air spaces within the lungs) and bronchitis.
- Smoking can also delay the healing of peptic ulcers and cause chronic pains in the legs – a condition called *claudication*. This can progress to gangrene and the need for amputation.
- Female smokers are likely to experience an early menopause.
- Middle-aged and elderly male smokers are likely to suffer from erectile dysfunction. Because smoking seems to sedate the sperm and reduce their motility, it can lower male fertility, too. This effect is reversed upon quitting.
- Osteoporosis – a disease in which the bones become weak and more prone to fractures – is accelerated in smokers.
- Smokers are two to six times more likely than non-smokers to have coughs, increased phlegm, wheezing and shortness of breath.
- Smokers have bad breath, stained teeth and maybe yellowed finger tips.
- The skin of a smoker becomes thin and more prone to wrinkling. The average smoker looks five years older than a non-smoker.
- Exercise tolerance is impaired by smoking.
- Female fertility is impaired by smoking, causing delays in conception after using oral contraceptives (see Chapter 8 for more information on oral contraceptives and high blood pressure).
- Smoking during pregnancy increases the risk of miscarriage, premature birth, light birth weight and death of the baby in its first year of life. The baby could also have abnormal brain development and a greater risk of SIDS (Sudden Infant Death Syndrome). Hyperactivity and behavioural problems can arise in a toddler.
- Children of parents who both smoke in the house obtain as

much nicotine as they would if they smoked 80 cigarettes a year –
hence they are called 'passive smokers'.

- The children of smokers are more likely to suffer from chronic
respiratory illnesses such as bronchitis, pneumonia and asthma.

Smoking and high blood pressure

As smoking can cause high blood pressure in susceptible people,
people who smoke are more likely than non-smokers to develop
high blood pressure and all its associated risks. In addition, a
smoker who already has high blood pressure is likely to see his or
her blood pressure rising further and eventually progress to heart
disease. A person's risk of developing heart disease increases alarm-
ingly in relation to the amount he or she smokes – i.e. someone
who smokes 40 a day stands a far greater chance of heart attack
than someone who smokes ten a day.

Nicotine is known as a *vaso-constrictor*, which means that it
narrows arteries and blood vessels, making it more difficult for
blood to move through the body. And as always when there is
damage to arteries and blood vessels, the heart must work harder
to pump blood through them, causing the heart muscle to become
over-developed (enlarged). Smoking also affects arteries and blood
vessels in the following ways:

- The carbon monoxide from smoking decreases levels of good
cholesterol (HDL) in the blood and raises levels of bad cholesterol (LDL), causing cholesterol deposits to form on blood vessel
walls. This gradually constricts the arteries and other blood
vessels, and once again the heart must work harder and faster to
push blood through.
- In smokers, a lack of oxygen in the body works with nicotine
to make the blood vessels too thin. When a blood vessel in the
heart bursts, the immediate outcome is a heart attack. When
a blood vessel in the head bursts, the immediate outcome is a
stroke.
- High levels of nicotine in the body can cause blood clots to form.
If immediate help is not sought, this often results in a heart
attack or stroke.

- Female smokers who also use oral contraceptives stand a far greater chance of developing high blood pressure than non-smokers who use oral contraceptives (see Chapter 8 for more information on this).

Some facts about smoking addiction

- Smoking is the main cause of preventable disease and death in the UK.
- 87 per cent of lung cancers are due to smoking.
- Most cases of emphysema and chronic bronchitis are due to smoking.
- There are 43 distinct cancer-causing chemicals in cigarettes.
- 30–40 per cent of all deaths from heart disease in the UK are directly related to smoking.
- The younger you are when you start smoking, the more likely you are to die prematurely from a smoking-related disease.
- People who smoke 20 a day die, on average, seven years earlier than people who have never smoked.
- People who smoke 20 a day stand more than double the risk of heart attack than non-smokers.
- Smokers who suffer a heart attack are more likely than non-smokers to die within an hour of the attack.
- One-third of smokers light their first cigarette within 30 minutes of getting up in the morning.
- One in 12 light up within the first five minutes.
- Nicotine is as addictive as heroin and cocaine.
- About 80 per cent of adult smokers started smoking before the age of 18.
- Only 2.5 per cent of smokers per year manage to quit for good.
- Most people try to quit several times before they succeed.
- A person who successfully stops smoking has the same risk of heart disease 15 years later as a lifelong non-smoker.
- Second-hand smoke can cause cancer in non-smokers. There are about 3,000 deaths per year from lung cancer in non-smokers.

What happens to your body when you stop smoking?

Health benefits accrue from the moment you refuse your next cigarette. However, when a drug the body has become accustomed to is no longer ingested, the body experiences a period of readjustment during which withdrawal symptoms take place. It is always best to know what symptoms to expect so you can prepare yourself to face them.

Withdrawal symptoms

When giving up smoking 'cold turkey', you are likely to experience restlessness, irritability, poor concentration, increased appetite, light-headedness, nocturnal waking and cravings. You might also have feelings of aggression and find yourself swinging in and out of depressions. It is normal for all of these symptoms to last for two to four weeks, with the exception of an increased appetite which can last two to three months. See p. 68 for more information on coping with withdrawal symptoms.

Prepare yourself for stopping smoking

Before you quit smoking, it's helpful to prepare yourself for what is to come. To do this, follow the advice below:

- Decide positively that you wish to quit, then write down your reasons for feeling this way. You need powerful reasons that will motivate you through the quitting process. As well as health reasons, you may wish to think about all the money you spend on smoking and all the time you waste taking cigarette breaks and going out to buy another pack.
- Before going to bed every night, repeat one of your reasons ten times.
- Try to understand why you smoke. For example, recognize that it creates a feeling of pleasure.
- Read up on the benefits of quitting.
- Set a date for smoking your last cigarette. Try to choose a day that is generally stress-free and that gives you the time to keep yourself busy. Ideally, the date should be within two weeks of reading this. If you smoke heavily at work, plan your quitting day for the start of a holiday period. By the time you return to work you should already be committed to quitting. Make your chosen quitting date sacred and don't let anything alter it. Plan to have an annual celebration of the day you gave up smoking.

- Before the day arrives, ask your doctor for advice regarding any health problems you have.
- Keep your expectations realistic and be aware that quitting is far from easy. At the same time, remember that millions of people worldwide quit smoking for good every year.
- Be aware that relapses are most likely in the first week after quitting, and be prepared. Use willpower, family, friends, the QUIT organization (see 'Useful addresses', p. 113) and any aids that help you through this critical period.
- If possible, find someone to quit with you. This could be a relative, friend or work colleague. Set your quitting date together and agree to support each other.
- Inform family and friends of your intentions and ask for their support.
- Warn the people around you that you may have some mood changes during the withdrawal period.
- As your quitting date approaches, rely most on the people who have already been supportive.
- Stay away from people who smoke. Most urges to start smoking again occur when a smoker is present.
- In the period leading up to your quitting date, start the exercise regime and healthy eating plan as described in Chapters 2 and 3. Exercise will help to relieve stress and provide you with more energy. Following a healthy eating plan should help you to conquer cravings and avoid weight gain.
- Get into the habit of drinking more fluids, getting plenty of rest and avoiding fatigue.
- Plan to avoid smoking triggers as much as possible. For instance, don't arrange to go for a drink with friends until the worst of your withdrawal symptoms are over. Make up your mind in advance to get up straight away after meals at home to clean your teeth or go for a walk – or you might plan to do a little sewing, sketching or something else that occupies your hands.
- Determine to follow a deep-breathing routine (as discussed in Chapter 5) whenever you experience cravings. A craving doesn't generally last for more than three to five minutes.
- If you always smoke when driving, plan to use public transport for a while.

- As occupying your hands may be a problem during the quitting process, make sure you always have a pen about your person, or buy a stress-relief aid to fiddle with.
- Contact QUIT and inform them that you intend to stop smoking. Their practical help, support and advice will be a boost, as will knowing that you can get in touch with them whenever you are struggling. (For details of QUIT, see 'Useful addresses', p. 113.)
- Believe you can quit if you persevere.

Ways to help you quit

To help you quit smoking, think of doing the following in the period before your planned quit date:

- Switch to a brand of cigarettes you don't like.
- Change to a low-tar low-nicotine brand – but at all costs avoid smoking more cigarettes than you were.
- Cut down the number of cigarettes you smoke.
- Postpone lighting your first cigarette for one hour each day.
- Decide in advance that you'll only smoke a certain number of cigarettes per day.
- Pour a glass of juice instead of a cigarette when you need a pick-me-up.
- Avoid smoking 'automatically'. Go to look at yourself in a mirror each time you light up – you may even decide you don't need that particular cigarette.
- Smoke only the cigarettes you really want.
- Wait until your cigarette pack is empty before you buy another.
- Don't carry cigarettes around with you. Make them difficult to get to.
- Don't empty your ashtrays. This will remind you of how many cigarettes you have smoked that day. Also, the smell will be distasteful.

Getting 'outside' help

There is plenty of help available for people who wish to quit smoking, as shown below:

- Get a free 'quit smoking' support pack and DVD from the NHS

Smoking Helpline website (see 'Useful addresses', p. 113, for more information). From this website you can download inspirational video-clips, a stop-smoking guide, an addiction test with advice for beating cravings and an information sheet.

- Visit your local NHS anti-smoking clinic at your doctor's surgery. Here group sessions are held by the practice nurse, quitting options are discussed and you will be given enough nicotine patches to last until the next session.

- Think about using nicotine replacement therapy in the form of chewing gum, skin patches, tablets, nasal spray or inhalers to ease withdrawal symptoms. Speak to your doctor or local pharmacist for information on which to try, and get some in before the big day.

On your quit date

Here is some important advice for when that big day arrives:

- Throw all your cigarettes and matches in the outside bin. Hide all your lighters and ashtrays.

- You might want to have your teeth cleaned at the dentist's to remove all the nicotine stains. Appreciate how nice they look and determine to keep them like that.

- Make a list of things you'd like to buy yourself and a few other special people, using the cash you would have spent on cigarettes. Now put your first week's cigarette money in a safe place and resolve to add that amount to it every week. Imagine how much you will have saved in six months.

- Chew on a toothpick or use a fake cigarette if you miss having something in your mouth.

- If you miss having something in your hands, play with a pen, paperclip or small ball.

- Avoid drinking tea, coffee and alcohol as you will associate these with smoking. Drink plenty of water, milk and fruit juices instead.

- Keep very busy all day. If you are not at work, take a long walk, go for a bike ride, to the swimming baths or even the cinema.

- Remind family and friends that this is your quit date and ask for their support.

- Do something special to celebrate the day, such as going for a massage or aromatherapy treatment, having your hair done, treating yourself to that book, film or play, or buying yourself a small gift such as flowers – you will be surprised at how you notice their perfume from now on.
- Recognize when you are rationalizing. For instance, if you catch yourself thinking, 'I'll just have one cigarette to soothe my nerves,' stop and think again! Remind yourself that there are better ways to relax, such as taking a bath or following a relaxation exercise.

In the days after you quit

In the days after you quit you can avoid temptation by doing the following:

- Make smoking difficult by starting new habits, such as taking up jogging, sketching, sewing, baking or solving crossword and sudoku puzzles.
- When your desire to smoke is intense, do something else such as performing your exercise routine, washing your hands, brushing your teeth, washing the dishes, styling your hair, giving yourself a manicure or walking the dog.
- Steer clear of situations in which you would normally smoke. If you must go to a gathering of people, stick with the non-smokers.
- Appreciate the clean taste in your mouth. Maintain it by regularly brushing your teeth and using a mouthwash. Understand that other people are not now smelling cigarettes on your breath.
- Get plenty of rest to counter extra activity. When resting, perform a relaxation routine and visualize yourself in a serene, restful place.
- Take more pride in your appearance.
- Congratulate yourself each time you get through a day without smoking. At the end of each week, reward yourself by buying yourself a treat or going out to the cinema or theatre.
- Use positive 'self-talk'. For instance, try repeating to yourself, 'I'm an intelligent person and I can do this,' 'I don't need to feel alone because everyone's behind me,' and 'I now know what to do in any situation, so there's nothing I can't deal with.'

When you feel desperate

- Keep oral substitutes handy for when you feel desperate. These could include dried fruit, pickled onions, raw carrots, apples, nuts, celery and sugarless gum.
- If you can, take a shower or bath.
- Take ten deep breaths and light a match while holding the last breath. Exhale slowly and blow out the match. Crush it in an ashtray as if it was a cigarette.
- Don't ever think that just one cigarette won't hurt. It will.

What happens to your body after you quit smoking

Within a few days of smoking your last cigarette your sense of smell and taste is likely to improve, you should be breathing more easily and your smoker's cough will not be as bad as it was. However, you may feel worse rather than better in yourself for a while because withdrawal symptoms are taking hold – but these are an important part of your recovery process which signal the beginning of a healthier life. They arise because your body is very quickly ridding itself of nicotine. If you didn't undergo withdrawal symptoms the nicotine would remain in your body and continue to increase your chances of dying prematurely from a cruel disease.

Help for particular symptoms

Here are some things you can do to lessen the impact of certain symptoms:

- *Dry mouth and sore throat* Chew chewing gum or fruit gums, sip on iced water or fruit juice.
- *Headaches* Use the relaxation technique as discussed in Chapter 5, take a warm bath with a few drops of lavender oil in it, brew a pot of wild lettuce tea.
- *Insomnia* Avoid coffee, tea, chocolate and alcohol after 6 p.m. Get up and read a boring book until you feel sleepy. Use the relaxation technique in Chapter 5.
- *Fatigue* Take regular naps. Try to fill your time, but don't push yourself as your body is already working hard, ridding itself of nicotine.

- *Hunger* Drink plenty of low-calorie liquids and stick to the healthy diet as discussed in Chapter 3. Eat dried fruit, nuts, raw fruit and cereal bars as snacks.
- *Feeling tense* Go for a walk, soak in a bath with lavender oil, use the relaxation technique as discussed in Chapter 5.
- *Constipation* Stick to the diet discussed in Chapter 3, eating plenty of fruit, vegetables and wholegrain cereals.

Dealing with temptation

In your first weeks as a non-smoker, the key to ongoing success is to avoid giving in to your urge to smoke – because you surely will be tempted at times. Whenever you crave a cigarette, ask yourself the following:

- Where am I?
- What am I doing?
- Who am I with?
- What was I just thinking?

You will soon see that the urge to smoke hits you at predictable times, so you must anticipate these times and find ways to get through them. Go back to the section headed 'Prepare yourself for stopping smoking' on p. 63 and re-read your reasons for quitting.

If you relapse

If you do smoke again, don't be too hard on yourself. Recognize that you've had a slip, see it as a small setback and immediately get back on track. It's important to identify the reason for the slip and work out how to cope if that particular set of circumstances happens again. Many smokers are worried about gaining weight if they quit, but this isn't inevitable. You can avoid weight gain by trying to stick to the healthy eating regime outlined in Chapter 3. Surely, though, a small weight gain – if it happens – is not a bad exchange for doing something that will so drastically improve your health? The extra weight is usually lost when the struggle to stop smoking is behind you and you are more able to devote yourself to healthy eating.

Some people may need professional help in the fight against

smoking. If you think this is what you require, your doctor should be able to provide extra motivation, and you may be prescribed nicotine gum or patches to get you over the worst period. If you think quitting is just too difficult, there are now tablets called bupropion (Zyban) which can help an addicted smoker resist the temptation to smoke.

5

Stress

Stress is the feeling we get when we are unable to deal with excessive mental or emotional pressure. It can comprise of anxiety, irritability, frequent headaches, palpitations, a feeling of isolation from family and friends, poor sleep and even depression. Unfortunately, many people who are stressed 'self-medicate' in the form of alcohol, smoking, over-eating and becoming less active than normal – but sadly, doing just one of these things can worsen the situation, the result being high blood pressure and its associated risks.

There is plenty of evidence to show that stress can cause a dramatic increase in blood pressure for as long as the individual feels that way. A person whose blood pressure was normal beforehand will be likely to see it return to normal once the stressor disappears, but each spike in blood pressure can cause damage to the blood vessels, heart and kidneys. It's also a fact that the cumulative damage occurring in a person who is regularly stressed is similar to that caused by long-term high blood pressure.

The stress response

Since the days of the ancient hunter-gatherer, the human body has produced extra quantities of the hormone *cortisol* – known as 'the stress hormone' – as a reaction to a perceived threat or a dangerous situation. Because the purpose of cortisol is to prepare the body to either fight or run away – this is known as 'the fight or flight response' – it was very useful thousands of years ago when people were faced with something like a charging wild animal. Sadly, our bodily makeup has changed very little over the years, which means that we perceive the pressures of modern living such as speaking in public, being stuck in traffic, divorce and redundancy in just the same way. The sudden rise in cortisol makes us aware that we are stressed, for our hearts begin beating faster and we feel very tense and 'wound up'. What we are not so aware of is that our blood pressure has shot up, and will stay up for as long as we are stressed.

The modern definition of stress is the state of mental or emotional tension resulting from adverse or very demanding circumstances. Some people are clearly more prone to getting stressed than others, which suggests they are less successful than others at controlling the stress response. In order to control the stress response adequately, it is necessary to be adept at the following:

- identifying events that trigger the stress response
- knowing how best to respond
- knowing the appropriate level of response
- knowing when to terminate the response.

Long-term stress

Cortisol is a vital part of the body's response to a troublesome situation, for it stimulates a reduced awareness of pain, heightened memory and a burst of energy. However, the rise in cortisol levels is not sufficiently helpful on its own. Indeed, it's equally important that the body's 'relaxation response' is quickly activated (see p. 75 for more information on relaxation). As we know, though, many individuals are not able to relax easily, and when that flaw is combined with the high-stress culture we live in, the stress response may be activated so frequently that the body has no time to return to normal in between times. This creates a situation of chronic stress, which in turn is likely to cause chronic high blood pressure with the risk of eventual arterial damage and cardiovascular disease or stroke.

Stress management strategies

Learning stress management strategies is a good means of handling stress. It is also possible to make certain lifestyle changes which stop your body from reacting to stress in the first place.

Here are some things you can do to lower your stress levels:

- Listen to music. Music is a great tension-reliever and can lower blood pressure, relax the body and calm the mind. For the best results, choose the music you most enjoy listening to.

- Listen to a radio comedy podcast. Radio podcasts can be down-loaded from a computer on to an iPod or MP3 player, and they are free from the BBC radio website. Laughter is a great way to dissipate stress.
- Watch a funny film on TV or DVD.
- Write down your thoughts in a diary. Putting down the things that stress you on paper can make them seem less of a problem and can help you to see solutions.
- Try to get plenty of sleep. (See p. 77 for more information on sleep and p. 79 for insomnia.)
- Carry out a deep breathing exercise, followed by a relaxation exercise and visualization (see pp. 75–6).
- Put a few drops of lavender oil in the bath and have a good soak.
- Treat yourself to one of the more relaxing complementary thera-pies (see Chapter 6).
- Use positive self-talk (see p. 80).
- Sing a jolly song loudly and with gusto to release tension. If you are too self-conscious to do this when there are people around, do it while you are having a shower. Singing alone while driving the car is a good stress reliever, too.
- Keep your living or working space tidy. Research has shown that a cluttered environment is emotionally draining and can cause additional stress.
- Simplify your daily routine. If you feel rushed all the time, alter your daily schedule so you spend less time on time-consuming activities that are not very important to you.
- Cultivate a supportive circle of friends. Friends you can really talk to and lean on in times of need are like gold dust, so hang on to them! Friends who take instead of giving will only drain you and make you feel more stressed, so it's best to gently drop them from your life.
- Learn to say 'no'. When people ask you to do something that you know will cause you stress, it's important to be able to say 'no'.
- Look on the bright side. When faced with a problem, try not to feel overwhelmed and resist the tendency to complain. Instead, focus your mind on finding solutions.
- Try to accept what you can't change. If you have made all the

recommended changes to your lifestyle and your blood pressure remains stubbornly high, don't blame yourself – you have done all you can. Unfortunately, some people can only lower their blood pressure by taking medication.

Exercise is a natural stress-buster which can reduce your systolic blood pressure by up to 10 mm Hg. You should, therefore, find it worthwhile to carry out some of the following activities:

- Go for a brisk walk.
- Carry out your chosen exercise routine (as discussed in Chapter 2). Remember that your doctor must give the go-ahead beforehand.
- Try yoga or Pilates. Either attending a yoga or Pilates class or using a DVD to do it at home is a great way to reduce stress.
- Have sex with your partner. Making love with that special someone is a great stress-reliever.
- Do some gardening. The physical nature of digging, weeding and planting can be a wonderfully relaxing pastime. It also allows your body to absorb fresh air and vitamin D, both of which help to reduce stress.
- Have fun with your children, grandchildren and/or nieces and nephews. Playful interaction with children is far more rewarding than simply supervising their activities. It lowers stress levels, too. Roll around on the carpet or lawn with them, kick a ball to each other or finger-paint a masterpiece together. Older children can be great companions for when you go shopping or to the cinema, and so on.

Using deep breathing to handle stress

In normal breathing, we take oxygen from the atmosphere down into our lungs. The diaphragm contracts and air is pulled into the chest cavity. When we breathe out, we expel carbon dioxide and other waste gases back into the atmosphere. But when we are stressed or upset, we tend to use the rib muscles to expand the chest. We breathe more quickly, sucking in shallowly. This is good in a crisis as it allows us to obtain the optimum amount of oxygen in the shortest possible time, providing our bodies with the extra power needed to handle the emergency. Some people do tend to get stuck in chest-breathing mode, however, which can impact on their physical and emotional health, often causing hyperventilation, panic attacks, chest pains, dizziness and gastro-intestinal problems.

To test your breathing, ask yourself:

- How fast am I breathing as I am reading this?
- Am I pausing between breaths?
- Am I breathing with my chest or with my diaphragm?

A deep breathing exercise

The following deep breathing exercise should, ideally, be performed daily:

1 Lie down and make yourself comfortable in a warm room where you know you will be alone for at least half an hour.
2 Close your eyes and try to relax.
3 Gradually slow down your breathing, inhaling and exhaling as evenly as possible.
4 Place one hand on your chest and the other on your abdomen, just below your rib-cage.
5 As you inhale, allow your abdomen to swell upward (your chest should barely move).
6 As you exhale, let your abdomen flatten.

Give yourself a few minutes to get into a smooth, easy rhythm. As worries and distractions arise, don't hang on to them. Wait calmly for them to float out of your mind – then focus once more on your breathing.

When you feel ready to end the exercise, open your eyes. Allow yourself time to become alert before rolling on to one side and getting up. With practice, you will begin breathing with your diaphragm quite naturally – and in times of stress, you should be able to correct your breathing without too much effort.

A relaxation exercise

Relaxation is one of the forgotten skills in today's hectic world, but it can help to counter the effects of stress. It's advisable, therefore, that you learn at least one relaxation technique.

The following exercise is perhaps the easiest:

1 Lie down and make yourself comfortable in a place where you will not be disturbed. (Listening to restful music may help you relax.)
2 Begin to slow down your breathing, inhaling through your nose to a count of two.
3 Ensuring that the abdomen pushes outwards (as explained on p. 75), exhale to a count of four, five or six.

After a couple of minutes, concentrate on each part of your body in turn, starting with your right arm. Consciously relax each set of muscles, allowing the tension to flow right out . . . Let your arm feel heavier and heavier as every last remnant of tension seeps away . . . Follow this procedure with the muscles of your left arm, then the muscles of your face, your neck, your stomach, your hips, and finally your legs.

Visualization

At this point, visualization can be introduced into the exercise. As you continue to breathe slowly and evenly, imagine yourself surrounded, perhaps, by lush, peaceful countryside, beside a gently trickling stream – or maybe on a deserted tropical beach, beneath swaying palm fronds, listening to the sounds of the ocean, thousands of miles from your worries and cares. Let the warm sun, the gentle breeze, the peacefulness of it all wash over you . . .

The tranquillity you feel at this stage can be enhanced by repeating the exercise frequently – once or twice a day is best. With time, you should be able to switch into a calm state of mind whenever you feel stressed.

Meditation

Arguably the oldest natural therapy, meditation is the simplest and most effective form of self-help. Dr Herbert Benson of Harvard Medical School has been able to show that meditation can normalize blood pressure, the pulse rate and the level of stress hormones in the blood. He has proven, too, that it produces changes in brain wave patterns, showing less excitability and strengthening the immune system and endocrine system (hormones).

The unusual thing about meditation is that it involves 'letting go', allowing the mind to roam freely. Most of us are used to trying to control our thoughts – in our work, for example – so letting go is not so easy as it sounds.

It may help to know that people who regularly meditate say they have more energy, require less sleep, are less anxious and feel far 'more alive' than before they did so. Ideally, the technique should be taught by a teacher – but, as meditation is essentially performed alone, it can be learned alone with equal success.

Meditation may, to some people, sound a bit off-beat. But isn't it worth a try – especially when you can do it for free? Kick off those shoes and make yourself comfortable, somewhere you can be alone for a while. Now follow these simple instructions:

1 Close your eyes, relax, and practise the deep breathing exercise as described.
2 Concentrate on your breathing. Try to free your mind of conscious control.
3 Letting it roam unchecked, try to allow the deeper, more serene part of you to take over.
4 If you wish to go further into meditation, concentrate now on mentally repeating a 'mantra' – a certain word or phrase. It should be something positive, such as 'relax', 'I feel calm', 'I am feeling much better' or even 'I am special.'
5 When you are ready to finish, open your eyes and allow time to adjust to the outside world before getting to your feet.

The aim of mentally repeating a mantra is to plant positive thoughts into your subconscious mind. It is a form of hypnosis, except that this is self-hypnosis: you alone control the messages placed there.

Getting better sleep

Getting a good night's sleep is of great importance to every human being on the planet. It helps to restore energy, gives the joints and soft tissues a chance to rest and helps us to cope with stress arising in everyday life.

The following suggestions can help you to get better-quality sleep:

• As caffeine is a stimulant, reduce the daily amount of caffeine you consume in coffee, tea, cola drinks and chocolate. It is best not to take caffeine at all in the three or four hours before bedtime.

- Avoid eating for at least two hours before bedtime.
- If possible, use the bed and bedroom only for sleeping (and sex).
- Ensure that the bedroom heating is not too high. A cooler bedroom is more conducive to sleep.
- As routine is the best way to regulate your body clock, try to go to bed at the same time every night. The recommended amount of sleep is seven to eight hours per night for adults.
- A quiet period before bedtime helps you to feel calm and prepares you for sleep. For example, instead of watching a late-night action film, try reading a book (something gentle) or listening to soothing music.
- Have a warm bath, followed by a warm milky drink, before going to bed.
- Don't watch TV in the bedroom before trying to sleep.
- Turn your bedside clock around so you are not tempted to keep checking the time.
- If you can't prevent certain thoughts or ideas running around your mind, get up for a few minutes and write them down – you are then more likely to stop thinking about them.
- If sleep still evades you, try counting down from 301. If you forget which number you're on, just continue from the last number you remember. This strategy doesn't work for everyone, so if it isn't helping don't persevere.
- When you just can't get to sleep, don't start tossing and turning. Instead, get up, make yourself a warm milky drink and for half an hour try reading a book you find boring. For such occasions, perhaps you could keep a book on a subject that doesn't hold any particular interest for you – a recipe book, an encyclopaedia, a research paper or instructions for using certain household items.
- If you suspect that the medication you are taking interferes with your sleep, tell your doctor. There is likely to be an alternative drug he or she can prescribe.
- If you can't get enough sleep no matter what you try, ask your doctor to refer you to a sleep therapist.

Insomnia

A person who is able to sleep well will wake up feeling refreshed and ready to face the day. It isn't always this way, however – especially if you are stressed. The insomnia often linked with chronic (long-term) stress is defined as the chronic inability to fall asleep or experience uninterrupted sleep, and it can follow any of the patterns listed below. You may have periods of time where your body sticks to one particular pattern, then periods when it sticks to another. It is also possible for your sleep pattern to be different virtually every night.

- You can't get to sleep for two to three hours after going to bed.
- You go to sleep easily enough, but wake up in the early hours and have great difficulty going back to sleep.
- You wake up several times during the night, sometimes for short periods and sometimes for longer periods.
- You wake too early in the morning and can't get back to sleep.

Strategies for curing insomnia

There are several 'natural' strategies for encouraging a return to a good sleeping rhythm, but it might be an idea to also use tricyclic medication for up to three months. This will provide added help for getting a good night's sleep. Speak to your doctor about this.

It's possible to develop good sleep habits by doing the following (some of these suggestions were mentioned earlier in this chapter):

- Try not to nap during the day. If you feel you can't cope without a nap, don't sleep for more than half an hour. Naps can prevent you from feeling sleepy at bedtime.
- Hang heavy curtains to make the bedroom as dark as possible.
- Before trying to sleep, unwind by listening to music or a relaxation CD, reading or watching an unexciting programme on TV.
- Have a warm milky drink.
- Shortly before bedtime take a warm bath (preferably using relaxing aromatherapy oils, as discussed on p. 87).
- Go to bed when you feel sleepy, so long as it is not before 9.30 p.m.
- Ensure that your bed and bedroom are comfortably warm, but not over-heated.

- Wear a sleep mask to help you sleep soundly for longer periods of time.
- Wear earplugs to eliminate distracting noises.
- Make yourself comfortable in bed, breathing slowly and evenly into your diaphragm. Clear your mind and allow your thoughts to drift. Don't hold on to any one thought, but let them pass unchecked.
- Set your alarm for the same time every morning.

Try to avoid the following:

- caffeine drinks after 6 p.m.
- alcohol before bedtime
- eating, drinking or reading in bed
- engaging in animated conversation (or arguments) before bedtime
- napping during the day
- sitting up to watch TV for long periods, particularly in the evening.

Taking up the last point, sitting to watch TV for several hours during daytime and evening is a habit that can interfere with sleep. This is because TV provokes numerous emotional responses in rapid succession, quickening the heart rate and releasing chemicals (such as adrenaline) for no useful purpose. When these chemicals are produced naturally, we deal with the situation and our blood flow is returned to normal. However, when chemicals are induced second-hand – such as occurs when watching TV – they remain in the bloodstream, causing tension to linger.

Self-talk

The way we speak to ourselves has great bearing on our stress levels. When we analyse our thoughts, we are often surprised at their extreme negativity, but they must be examined before we can begin to change their destructive pattern. When the TV breaks down, for example, your initial thoughts may be, 'It's so unfair! I was really looking forward to watching that film!', 'This is all I need! I can't afford a new TV!', 'Even if it can be repaired, it will probably cost a small fortune!', 'What am I supposed to do with my time –

sit twiddling my thumbs?' – stress-provoking thoughts by any standard! However, by being aware that negative thoughts create stress, you can train yourself into more positive self-talk. Using the same example, you may, instead, think, 'I'll ring around for quotes in the morning. Maybe it won't cost much to repair', 'It was on its last legs anyway. I'll take the opportunity to buy a more up-to-date set', 'I'll look for a 0 per cent hire-purchase deal', 'I could buy a reconditioned TV if I can't afford a new one', 'I could rent one and not have to worry about repair costs', 'I wonder if my friend down the road is watching that film. I'll ring and ask if I can join her', or 'In the meantime, this is my chance to read that book, finish my model-painting, phone Aunt Jane . . .'

The following examples of stress-relieving self-talk can be applied to many potentially stressful situations:

'I'll break this problem into separate sections. They'll be easier to handle.'

'I'll take things one step at a time.'

'Is this really worth getting upset and angry over?'

'I've coped before, so I'll cope again.'

'I can always ask for help if I need it.'

'It could have been so much worse.'

'This is hardly a matter of life or death!'

'There's nothing I can do about this situation, so I'll have to accept it.'

Life stress evaluation

If you take time to evaluate all the relationships and activities in your everyday life, you are likely to find that some prompt more stress than benefit. High blood pressure demands that you protect your body and nourish your mind. 'Involvements' that have ceased to do this are probably harmful.

In reviewing your relationships and activities, however, remember that personal interactions and energy-related performances will always produce a certain amount of stress. It is when the stress outweighs the positive gains that you need to consider limiting or ceasing your involvement.

Coping with stress at work

A range of studies have indicated that there is a strong association between high blood pressure and psychological and psychosocial factors. Moreover, it seems that for people who already have high blood pressure, continued job strain can bring on angina (severe chest pain caused by insufficient blood supply to the heart) or even a heart attack – although the latter is quite rare.

The causes of job stress include the following:

- high job demands
- tight deadlines
- too little support
- excessive effort for little reward.

A 1999 government health white paper stated that people who are under a lot of stress at work are more likely than others to develop cardiovascular disease. Indeed, studies have shown that women in high stress–low control jobs are at more than 70 per cent risk of getting cardiovascular disease than women in jobs with high levels of control. Moreover, men in high stress–low control jobs are approximately 50 per cent more likely to develop cardiovascular disease than their counterparts in high control jobs.

When this is combined with poor diet and inactivity, for example, the risk of developing cardiovascular disease becomes even greater. It doesn't help that the good management of people is a very rare skill.

However, it's possible to cope better with job stress by doing the following:

- Incorporate physical activity into your day – e.g. walking up the stairs instead of taking the lift, and getting off the bus a stop earlier and walking the rest of the way.
- If you work in a very loud factory, make sure that you use the ear-defenders provided. Constant exposure to loud noise can cause stress as well as deafness and tinnitus.
- When stress overwhelms you, take a few minutes out to perform a deep-breathing exercise (see p. 75).
- Ask your manager for an assistant if your workload is too great.
- If you are being constantly harassed by your manager(s) to meet

deadlines and so on, explain that you have high blood pressure and ask if they could relax their demands somewhat.

- If there is nothing you can do about the pressure of your job, ask to be transferred to another department or look for another job.

6

Complementary therapies

An increasing number of people with health problems are turning to complementary therapies such as acupuncture, aromatherapy and so on, often used in conjunction with their mainstream drugs. If you are using or thinking of using complementary therapies, please be aware that some types can cause adverse reactions and their quality and strength is not controlled by a regulating body. In comparison with mainstream medicine, where a great deal of research has been carried out, there has been very little research and few controlled scientific trials into the effects of complementary medicine. If you decide to try a particular therapy, I would advise that you find out as much about it as you can beforehand. You could also ask your doctor's advice.

However, unlike mainstream drugs that are mainly composed of chemical compounds, complementary therapies are entirely natural comprising such things as touch, aroma, talk (suggestion) and the intake of natural compounds such as herbs. Nevertheless, such compounds can occasionally cause adverse reactions such as headaches and stomach upsets; in rare cases they can even provoke a more serious response such as thinning the blood, which leads to excessive bleeding.

It's interesting to note that many people who use complementary therapies report significant benefits. Perhaps some of the improvement they feel comes from knowing they are doing something positive to help themselves, but it has to be assumed that the therapies themselves are responsible for at least a part of the improvement.

There is no doubt that the more relaxing therapies can reduce the stress which often exacerbates high blood pressure.

Acupuncture

An ancient form of Oriental healing, acupuncture involves puncturing the skin with fine needles at specific points in the body. These points are located along energy channels (meridians) that are believed to be blocked in a person with health problems (see Figure 24).

This energy is known as *chi* (also spelt 'qi'). Needles are inserted to increase, decrease or unblock the flow of chi energy so that the balance of yin and yang is restored.

Yin, the female force, is calm and passive; it also represents dark, cold, swelling and moisture. On the other hand, yang, the male force, is stimulating and aggressive, representing heat, light,

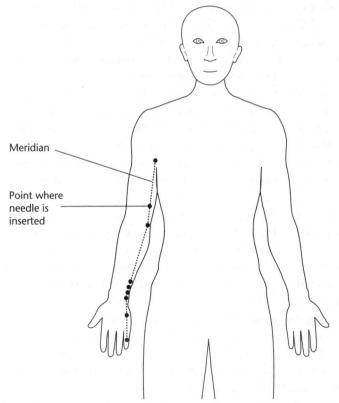

Meridian

Point where needle is inserted

Figure 24 Meridians and points where needles are inserted to relieve high blood pressure

contraction and dryness. It is thought that an imbalance in these forces is the cause of illness and disease. For example, a person who feels the cold and suffers fluid retention and fatigue would be considered to have an excess of yin. A person suffering from repeated headaches, however, will be deemed to have an excess of yang. Emotional, physical and environmental factors are believed to disturb the chi energy balance, and can also be treated. According to acupuncturists, following a healthy balanced diet, as recommended in Chapter 3, can go a long way towards restoring the balance of yin and yang, too.

In your acupuncture session, the therapist determines your particular acupuncture points – it is thought there are as many as 2,000 acupuncture points on the body and a set method is used to establish exactly where they are. At a consultation, questions may be asked about your lifestyle, sleeping patterns, fears, phobias and reactions to stress. Your pulses will be felt, after which the acupuncture itself is carried out, very fine needles being placed at the relevant sites. The first consultation will normally last for an hour, and your blood pressure readings should be reduced after four to six sessions – if not, there is really no point in carrying on.

Acupuncturists state that acupuncture is one of the most effective complementary means of lowering high blood pressure. It is said to work by blocking certain nerve pathways and stimulating particular hormone production. When conventional acupuncture is combined with electro-acupuncture – in which a device sends a pulsating electrical current into the acupuncture needles – acupuncturists claim that the effects on blood pressure are even more profound. In addition, they say that when several pairs of needles are used and the electric current passed from one needle to another, the excitatory response of the cardiovascular system is greatly reduced.

It is recommended that herbs such as Tian Ma (*Gastrodia rhizome*) and Xia Ku Cao (*Prunella*) are drunk three times a day as herbal tea infusions during the weeks of acupuncture treatment. This is believed to bring about the best result in reducing stress and bringing blood pressure down.

Aromatherapy

Certain health disorders are treated by stimulating our sense of smell with aromatic oils – known as *essential oils*. It is believed that such stimulation with a particular smell can help to treat a particular health problem. Indeed, there's no doubt at all that aromatherapy can aid relaxation and help to reduce the stress that is associated with rises in blood pressure.

Concentrated essential oils are extracted from plants and may be inhaled, rubbed directly into the skin or used in bathing. Each odour relates to its plant of origin – so lavender oil has the aroma of the lavender plant, and geranium has the aroma of the geranium plant.

Plant essences have been used for healing throughout the ages, smaller amounts being used for aromatherapy purposes than in herbal medicines. Aromatherapy oils are obtained either by steaming a particular plant extract until the oil glands burst, or by soaking the plant extract in hot oil so that the cells collapse and release their essence.

Techniques used in aromatherapy

There are several ways of using aromatherapy. The main ones are as follows:

- *Inhalation* Giving the fastest result, the inhalation of essential oils has a direct influence on the olfactory (nasal) organs, which is immediately received by the brain. Steam inhalation is the most popular technique, carried out either by mixing a few drops of oil with a bowlful of boiling water and leaning over it to breathe in the steam, or by using an oil burner, where the flame from a tea-light candle heats a small saucer of water containing a few drops of oil.
- *Massage* Essential oils produced specifically for massage are normally pre-diluted. They should never be applied to the skin in an undiluted (pure) form. When using undiluted essential oils, mix three or four drops with a neutral carrier oil, such as olive oil, tea tree oil or safflower oil. After penetrating the skin, the oils are absorbed by the body, and this is believed to exert a positive influence on a particular organ or set of tissues. Massage

is helpful in easing sore muscles, increasing circulation and relaxing tension.

- *Bathing* Tension and anxiety can be reduced by using aroma-therapy oils in the bath. A few drops of pure essential oil should be added directly to running tap water – it mixes more efficiently this way. No more than 20 drops of oil in total should be used.

Oils for relaxation

Lavender is the most popular oil for relaxation purposes. It is known to be a wonderful restorative and excellent for relieving tension headaches as well as stress. However, there are several others that used either alone or blended can provide a relaxing atmosphere – Roman chamomile and ylang ylang, for example. Ylang ylang has relaxing properties and a calming effect on the heart rate, and can relieve palpitations and raised blood pressure. Chamomile can be very soothing, too, and aids both sleep and digestion.

Drop your relaxation oils into the vessel part of an oil burner and top up with water. Light a tea-light candle (placed beneath the burner) and try to relax while the essential oils scent the whole room and you inhale their fragrance. Such oils are safe around babies and children as, rather than being overpowering, the aroma is soft and soothing.

Recipe 1

- 5 drops of lavender
- 2 drops of Roman chamomile
- 1 drop of ylang ylang.

Blend well and diffuse in a burner.

Recipe 2

- 8 drops of mandarin
- 3 drops of neroli
- 3 drops of ylang ylang.

Blend well and diffuse in a burner.

Recipe 3

- 10 drops of bergamot
- 2 drops of rose otto
- 3 drops of Roman chamomile.

Blend well and diffuse in a burner.

Relaxation recipes 2 and 3 can be added to 50 cc (just under 2 fl oz) of distilled water, shaken well and used in a spray bottle for a non-toxic room-freshener with relaxing properties.

Recipe 4

For relaxation, this is a great blend for use in the bath.

- 3 drops of lavender
- 2 drops of marjoram
- 2 drops of basil
- 1 drop of vetiver
- 1 drop fennel.

Oils for lowering blood pressure

Aromatherapy experts believe that clary sage, marjoram, melissa, lavender and ylang ylang essential oils can lower high blood pressure. These five oils are of most benefit when used to massage the body, and can be used alone or in any combination.

Essential oils to avoid

People with high blood pressure should be aware that the following essential oils are very stimulating and should therefore be avoided:

- hyssop
- rosemary
- sage
- thyme.

If you are planning to have an aromatherapy massage, it's important to tell the therapist that you have high blood pressure and have been advised to avoid the above-mentioned oils.

Hypnotherapy

Hypnotherapy is commonly described as an altered state of consciousness, lying somewhere between being awake and being asleep. People under hypnosis are aware of their surroundings, yet their minds are, to a large extent, under the control of the hypnotist. The main purposes of hypnotherapy are to promote relaxation, reduce tension, increase energy and boost motivation. It also aims to increase confidence and make a person more able to cope with problems.

At a hypnotherapy session, the therapist will take a full psychological and physiological history, then slowly talk you into a trance state. Once you are in that altered state of consciousness with a more receptive state of mind, the therapist may begin to explore the root cause of any problematic cause of tension and anxiety. Another tactic he or she may use is 'direct suggestion' – e.g. intimating that you will in future react more calmly in certain situations, or planting the thought in your head that you hate the taste and smell of cigarettes. Of course, the exact nature of the therapy depends largely on the problem for which treatment is being sought.

One common fear is that while the patient is in a trance the therapist may implant dangerous suggestions or extract improper personal information. I can only say that patients can come out of a trance at any time – particularly if they are asked to do or say anything they would not even contemplate when awake. And malpractice would only have to be brought to light once to ruin the therapist's career. You may prefer to visit a hypnotherapist recommended by your doctor.

There are many anecdotal reports of improvements from using hypnotherapy, but many experts say there is insufficient scientific evidence for them to promote this type of treatment. It is definitely an area worthy of further research, and it is to be hoped this takes place in years to come.

In the meantime, lots of people have used hypnotherapy with great success to help them stop smoking, to overcome a phobia, to eat or drink less or react more calmly to stressful situations. If you have high blood pressure and have any of the above-mentioned problems, I would say that hypnotherapy is well worth a try.

Homeopathy

The homeopathic approach to medicine is holistic – the overall health of a person, physical, emotional and psychological, is assessed before treatment commences. The practitioner will ask you about your medical history and personality traits, then offer a remedy compatible with your symptoms as well as with your temperament and characteristics. Consequently, two individuals with the same disorder may be offered entirely different remedies.

The homeopathic concept is that 'like cures like'. It is said that the full healing abilities of homeopathy were first recognized in the early nineteenth century when German doctor Samuel Hahnemann noticed that the herbal cure for malaria – which was based on an extract of cinchona bark (quinine) – actually produced symptoms of malaria. Further tests convinced him that the production of mild symptoms caused the body to fight the disease. He went on to successfully treat malaria patients with dilute doses of cinchona bark.

Each homeopathic remedy is first 'proved' by being taken by a healthy person – usually a volunteer homeopath – and the symptoms noted. This remedy is said to be capable of curing the same symptoms in an ill person. The whole idea of 'proving' and using homeopathic remedies can be difficult to comprehend, as it is exactly the opposite of how conventional medicines operate.

Although the remedies are safe and non-addictive, occasionally the patient's symptoms may worsen briefly. This is known as a 'healing crisis' and is usually short-lived. It is actually a good indication that the remedy is working well.

Case studies suggest that homeopathy can bring significant relief for most health problems; however, to date no convincing clinical research studies exist. A range of remedies can be found in most high-street chemists and on-line homeopathic chemists.

The remedies often used in treating high blood pressure are as follows:

- *Nux vomica* for people with high blood pressure and irritable fatigue caused by lack of sleep, stress or overwork. Tense muscles, feeling chilled, joint pain and indigestion are symptoms. Take the 30C strength twice daily for up to 14 days. Repeat the dose if beneficial.

- *Argentums nitricum* for people whose blood pressure rises with anxiety and nervousness. Their anticipation of stressful events brings on dizziness, headache, diarrhoea and pounding pulses.
- *Aurum metallicum* for serious people who are focused on their career and accomplishments, whose blood pressure problems are mostly related to stress. When they feel they have made a mistake, they react by worrying, being depressed or having flares of anger.
- *Calcarea carbonica* for people with high blood pressure who tire easily and have little stamina. They are responsible in nature, but feel overwhelmed when ill and worry about having a nervous breakdown.
- *Glonoinum* for people with high blood pressure who experience pounding headaches and visible throbbing in the blood vessels of the neck. Their chests can feel congested or hot, and they feel worse for moving around, after drinking alcohol and after heat and sun exposure.
- *Lachesis* for people with high blood pressure who are intense, passionate, talkative and whose agitation makes them feel like a pressure cooker. They may have a great fear of disease and often feel suspicious, vengeful or jealous.
- *Phosphorous* for people with high blood pressure who are sensitive, suggestible and sympathetic. They have a tendency towards feeling weak, 'spaced out' and dizzy.
- *Sanguinaria* for people with high blood pressure who feel that blood is rushing to their heads. They tend to have flushed cheeks, pulsing in the neck, headaches, migraines, right-sided neck and shoulder problems, allergies, heartburn and digestive problems.

Some important advice if you wish to self-treat

It's recommended that you only self-treat in conditions where you are not able to see a qualified homeopath, such as when you are on holiday and have eaten all the wrong foods and drunk a lot of alcohol, or if you have begun smoking again during a particularly stressful work-related assignment that has taken you away from home. Choose the remedy which most closely matches your personality and symptoms and use a low-potency preparation such as

6X, 6C, 12X, 12C, 30X or 30C. Follow the label instructions very carefully.

Qualified homeopaths study their 'trade' in great depth over six long years. This is why simply following a few personality and symptom indicators is hardly adequate when it comes to selecting the most appropriate herbal remedy and knowing how to judge its success or failure.

You should certainly not even think of self-treating after encountering symptoms such as severe headache, dizziness, blurred vision and nausea, for these are indicators that your blood pressure is far too high. In this instance, you should seek urgent medical attention.

If you are satisfied that you are self-treating in the right conditions (see p. 92), take one dose only and wait for a response. Should you experience improvement, it's best to wait a little longer to get the best from the remedy. If the improvement is only slight or has clearly stopped, you may take another dose. Some people need to take a dose several times an hour and others only once a day – it is dependent upon the individual, and everyone is different. Of course, if you see no improvement at all within a reasonable length of time, stop taking it and either select a different remedy or wait until you can see a qualified homeopath.

Biofeedback

Biofeedback is a treatment technique in which people can improve physical and emotional problems by using signals from their own bodies. Physiotherapists use biofeedback to help stroke victims regain movement in paralysed muscles and psychologists use it to help anxious clients learn to relax.

In the late 1960s, when the term *biofeedback* was first coined, research showed that certain involuntary actions like heart rate, blood pressure and brain function can be altered by tuning into the body. For instance, many people calm anxiety by reading an interesting book. As a result, their heart stops racing and their blood pressure drops to more normal levels. Later research showed that biofeedback can help in the treatment of many conditions and that we have more control over so-called involuntary function than we once thought possible. Scientists are currently trying to determine just how much voluntary control we can exert.

Biofeedback is now widely used to treat pain, high and low blood pressure, paralysis, epilepsy and many other disorders. The technique is taught by psychiatrists, psychologists, doctors and physiotherapists.

If you have a health problem that is exacerbated by stress, a biofeedback specialist will normally teach you:

- how to use a relaxation technique;
- how to identify the circumstances that trigger (or worsen) your symptoms;
- how to cope with events you have previously avoided because of your symptoms;
- how to set attainable goals;
- how to regain control of your life.

In using biofeedback, you must learn to examine your day-to-day life in order to ascertain whether you are somehow contributing to your health problem. You must recognize that you can, by your own efforts, get far more out of your life. In the correct use of biofeedback, bad habits must be changed and, most importantly, you must accept much of the responsibility for maintaining your own health.

Scientists believe that relaxation is the key to the success of this technique. You will be taught to react with a calmer frame of mind to certain stimuli – being asked to look after a young child when you feel tired already, for example. As a result, the stress response is not triggered and cortisol and other stress hormones are not pumped into the bloodstream. Without biofeedback training, cortisol and so on may be released repeatedly, giving rise to chronic anxiety, stress, muscle tension and depression. However, with biofeedback training, it is easier to say 'no' or to take any other action necessary to protect yourself and improve your condition.

If you think you might benefit from biofeedback training, discuss the matter with your doctor.

Reflexology

Reflexology, an ancient Oriental therapy, was only recently adopted in the Western world. It operates on the proposition that the body is divided into different energy zones, all of which can be exploited in the prevention and treatment of any disorder.

Reflexologists have identified ten energy channels, beginning in the toes and extending to the fingers and the top of the head. Each channel relates to a particular bodily zone, and to the organs in that zone. For example, the big toe relates to the head – the brain, ears, sinus area, neck, pituitary glands and eyes. By applying pressure to the appropriate terminal in the form of a small, specialized massage, a practitioner can determine which energy pathways are blocked.

Experts in this type of manipulative therapy claim that all the organs of the body are reflected in the feet. They also believe that reflexology aids the removal of waste products and blockages within the energy channels, improving circulation and lymph gland function. Reflexology is certainly relaxing – for the mind as well as the body. Indeed, as well as reducing stress, it can improve depression.

Many therapists prefer to take down a full case-history before commencing treatment. Each session takes up to 45 minutes (the preliminary session may take longer), and you will be treated sitting in a chair or lying down.

Herbal remedies

Herbal medicine is the oldest system of medicine available and remains the most widely used. Indeed, according to the World Health Organization, 80 per cent of the world's population use herbalism as their main form of treatment.

Your chosen trained herbalist will normally check your pulse rate and the colour of your tongue for clues as to which bodily organs are energy-depleted. He or she will then write a prescription for very precise doses according to your needs. Tablets made from compressed herbal extracts are often given, but you may simply receive a bag of weighed and ground dried roots, flowers and bark from which you should make an infusion according to the herbalist's instructions. Herbal nerve tonics and stress-reducing adaptogens are particularly supportive of the nervous system in people with stress-related disease.

If you wish to self-prescribe two or three herbal remedies, choose from the list below, according to your particular health problem. Always use herbal remedies with caution, and inform your doctor before starting treatment as they can interact with your prescription medications.

- *Hawthorn* Studies have shown that some patients taking a hawthorn supplement have a reduction in diastolic blood pressure after three or four months.
- *Mistletoe* This herb is said to contain active substances that normalize the whole cardiovascular system, effectively soothing and strengthening the heart. It is therefore said to be invaluable for reducing high blood pressure.
- *Cayenne* This herb is second only to garlic for its ability to lower blood pressure. For best results, use hot peppers such as Mexican or Thai (serranos, habeñeros and African bird peppers) rather than jalapeños.
- *Garlic* In a study of four controlled trials into the effects of garlic powder supplements, it was found that in three there was a significant reduction in systolic blood pressure, and in all of them there was a reduction in diastolic blood pressure. Researchers concluded, therefore, that garlic powder supplements may be of benefit in treating mild high blood pressure. Please note that as garlic can thin the blood and interact with many drugs and supplements (such as warfarin, pentoxifylline, aspirin, vitamin E and *Ginkgo biloba*), garlic powder supplements should only be taken under the supervision of your doctor.
- *Red clover* This herb is great for thinning the blood and can therefore decrease high blood pressure. Ensure that you are given the blossoms when they are a rich purple colour rather than brown, which would mean they were picked when dying or dead.
- *Ginkgo biloba* This herbal antioxidant is useful for improving blood circulation. As a result, cognitive function (concentration, memory, etc.) is improved, as is energy production. As people

taking prescription medication such as warfarin and aspirin can react adversely to this supplement, please consult your doctor before use. Also, if you are taking the herb white willow bark for a pain condition, you should avoid *Ginkgo biloba*.

- *St John's wort* This herb is probably the most successful natural antidepressant in the world. It works by increasing the action of the chemical serotonin, improving sleep and benefiting the immune system. If you think you are suffering from depression, this may be an effective treatment. However, antidepressants prescribed by your doctor are often more beneficial.

- *Rhodiola rosea* This powerful nutrient belongs to the family of adaptogenic herbs, which encourage the body to adapt to stress. Research has shown that *Rhodiola rosea* has a protective effect on the immune system, helps to raise energy levels and aids detoxi-fication. It also has revitalizing properties and helps to stabilize mood swings. Follow the dosage instructions on the label.

- *Ashwagandha* Also an adaptogenic herb, ashwagandha (some-times called Indian ginseng) is an important tonic, containing a broad range of healing powers that are rare in the plant kingdom. Not only is it good for boosting energy levels, it has also been shown in research to help rejuvenate the nervous system, enhance memory and concentration and ease insomnia and stress. Follow the dosage instructions on the label.

- *Siberian ginseng* This adaptogenic herb helps to increase physical endurance under stress, protects against infections and improves hormone activity. Take 4–8 g of dried root, or 20–40 ml for tinc-ture, or 4–8 drops of fluid extract or 200–400 mg of solid extract daily.

7

Medications

The target of all blood pressure treatments is to reduce blood pressure to at least 140/90. This figure is lowered to 130/80 if you already have heart disease or have suffered a stroke, or if you have kidney disease or diabetes. Unfortunately, using natural means alone – such as eating the right foods, reducing salt and alcohol intake, getting regular exercise and stopping smoking – does not always have sufficient effect, making it essential that you discuss blood pressure medications with your doctor.

Keep in mind, though, that using drug therapy is not an indication of failure on your part: it simply means that the steps you have taken are not quite enough on their own. Don't, at all costs, be tempted to revert to your old lifestyle. This would mean taking a higher drug dosage than you would need if you were also making positive changes to your lifestyle. In other words, if you need to take medication for your blood pressure, it's important that you also continue to make the lifestyle changes discussed in this book.

There are five main classes of drugs to lower blood pressure, and in each class there are several types and brands of drug. These are:

- ACE inhibitors
- angiotensin receptor blockers (or ARBs)
- calcium channel-blockers
- beta-blockers
- diuretics.

ACE inhibitors

ACE inhibitors (the ACE stands for *angiotensin converting enzyme*) usually have names that end in 'pril', such as ramipril, cilazapril, captopril, enalapril, lisinopril, fisinopril, perindopril, trandolapril and quinapril. They are medicines that help to block the production of a hormone called *angiotensin II,* which normally works on blood vessel walls to make them narrower. When angiotensin II flows unchallenged through the body, the narrowed vessels mean blood has less space in which to move, causing blood pressure to go up. A drug which inhibits the action of angiotensin II, however, causes the blood vessels to relax and dilate, and so blood pressure goes down.

ACE inhibitors have the additional function of reducing the amount of fluid reabsorbed by the kidneys, which also helps to lower blood pressure. People who have heart failure or diabetic kidney disease or who have already suffered a heart attack find particular benefit from taking this kind of medication.

ACE inhibitors should not be taken by individuals with certain kinds of artery problems and/or in pregnancy. There are usually no side effects, but some people are left with a persistent cough.

The kidneys

Before prescribing ACE inhibitors, your doctor will take a blood test to check that your kidneys are functioning normally. The blood test will be repeated two weeks after commencing the drug and within two weeks of any change in dosage. It is then usual for an annual blood test to be carried out.

The kidneys are intricately involved in the pressure of blood flow (blood pressure) because they control the amount of fluid retained in the blood versus the amount lost as waste in the urine. High blood pressure can damage the small blood vessels in the kidneys, making them unable to filter waste from the blood (in the form of urine). When kidney damage is evident or thought to be a likely future occurrence, a doctor will often prescribe ACE inhibitors to protect the kidneys, rather than prescribing other blood pressure medications that will reduce blood pressure equally well but will not have a protective effect on the kidneys.

The National Heart, Lung, and Blood Institute (NHLBI), one of the US National Institutes of Health, recommends that people with diabetes or impaired kidney function keep their blood pressure below 130/80.

Angiotensin receptor blockers

There are several types of angiotensin receptor blockers (ARBs, also known as *angiotension II receptor antagonists*), and they all have names ending in 'sartan'. Examples are candesartan, eprosartan, olmesartan, valsartan, telmisartan, irbesartan and losartan.

ARBs work in a similar way to ACE inhibitors in that they block the effects of the hormone angiotensin II. This can be of great benefit to a person with high blood pressure as angiotensin II triggers a hormone that makes the body retain fluid, and having more fluid in your body – i.e. in a restricted space – causes blood pressure to rise. ARBs lower blood pressure by causing the blood vessels to relax and widen, which makes it far easier for blood to flow through. In addition, they reduce the amount of fluid retained by the body, which also brings down the pressure of blood flow. As a result, they are a popular first-choice medication for high blood pressure. They are also the medication of choice for people who are under 55 and not of Afro-Caribbean origin. People who have kidney disease or diabetes as well as high blood pressure are often prescribed this type of drug, as there is evidence to show ARBs can protect the kidneys. Like other blood pressure medications, ARBs must be taken on a long-term basis. They can cause dizziness as a side effect.

You should not take ARBs if you are pregnant, breastfeeding or planning a pregnancy. Any side effects linked to this type of medication are usually mild and short-lived. The most common side effects are dizziness, headache and cold- or flu-like symptoms. In rare instances, an individual can have an allergic reaction to an ARB, causing swelling around the mouth and throat, and breathing difficulties. If this happens to you, contact your doctor for immediate help.

ARBs are more efficient at lowering blood pressure if you also reduce the amount of salt you consume.

Calcium channel-blockers

The term *calcium channel-blockers* refers to a group of drugs which reduce the amount of calcium entering particular muscle cells. In high blood pressure, blocking calcium in this way causes the muscle cells to relax. This has the effect of widening the arteries and lowering blood pressure. Calcium channel-blockers are particularly helpful for a person with angina pains, for they widen the coronary arteries and so ease the pain.

The calcium channel-blocker verapamil is commonly used to treat angina and high blood pressure. It can also regulate an abnormally fast heartbeat (a condition called *arrhythmia*), which it does by stopping calcium from entering special conducting cells in the heart. A person with arrhythmia should not take verapamil in combination with a beta-blocker drug.

Diltiazem, another calcium channel-blocker, is also used to treat angina and high blood pressure – but not arrhythmia. It is therefore often prescribed in addition to a beta-blocker drug. As they effectively relax the heart, neither verapamil nor diltiazem should be used if you have heart failure.

There is also the dihydropyridine group of calcium channel-blockers with names all ending in 'ipine'. They include lacidipine, amlodipine, lercanidipine, felodipine, nifedipine, nicardipine and nimodipine. These drugs effectively relax the blood vessels but are less useful at relaxing the heart muscle than verapamil or diltiazem. Apart from lacidipine, lercanidipine and isradipine, this group of calcium channel-blockers is used to treat high blood pressure and angina. Lacidipine, lercanidipine and isradipine are prescribed only for high blood pressure. Dihydropyridine calcium channel-blockers are not beneficial for treating arrhythmia and, like verapamil, can worsen heart failure. This type of drug can be taken in combination with a beta-blocker drug. Indeed, the combination is often used to ease angina pains when either a dihydropyridine calcium channel-blocker or beta-blocker is ineffective in isolation.

Calcium channel-blockers are usually side-effect free, but may occasionally cause flushing and a headache, which should ease within a few days of starting the tablets. In some people, dihydropyridine calcium channel-blockers can cause mild swelling in the ankles. Constipation is fairly common, too, particularly with verapamil. This can be assuaged by increasing the amount of fibre you eat and drinking more fluids. However, as grapefruit juice can interact with calcium channel-blockers, it should be avoided.

You should consult a doctor if you wish to stop taking a calcium channel-blocker, as sudden withdrawal can cause a rebound flare-up of angina.

Beta-blockers

When a natural hormone called *noradrenaline* enters special receptors in the arteries and heart, the arteries become narrow and the heart beats faster. So why is noradrenaline released? It occurs in response to one or more nerves being stimulated by adrenaline, which rushes into the bloodstream from the adrenal glands when the individual is frightened or anxious. Someone who is very tense, nervous and/or excitable is likely to have an excess of noradrenaline in his or her bloodstream on a fairly constant basis, causing high blood pressure and all of its risks.

Beta-blockers have been produced to prevent these things happening. They work by blocking the action of noradrenaline, as a result of which blood pressure is reduced and there is no longer any need for the heart to beat faster. High blood pressure, angina pains, arrhythmias and heart failure are treated by beta-blockers, as well as some of the symptoms caused by anxiety.

The possible side effects associated with beta-blockers include depression, tiredness, vivid dreams, impotence, wheezing, indigestion, cold hands and feet and fainting – although all of these things are rare. Faintness can occur when the heart rate slows too much, probably because the dosage you are taking is too high. If you experience any troublesome symptoms, you should speak to your doctor.

Beta-blockers have names that end in 'lol'. Examples are atenolol, esmolol, nadolol, acebutolol, carvedilol, betaxolol, sotalol, pindolol, metoprolol, celiprolol, labetalol and oxprenolol. They are often prescribed in combination with diuretics or calcium channel-blockers. Beta-blockers should not be withdrawn suddenly as the result can be palpitations, a rise in blood pressure and/or the onset of angina pains. Your doctor will advise a gradual reduction in dose.

Diuretics

Often called 'water tablets', diuretics act on the kidneys to raise the levels of salt and water that exit the body in the urine. As a result, more urine than normal is passed. It's important that excess salt is removed from the body – otherwise it would cause too much fluid to build up in the blood vessels, which would raise the person's blood pressure. When the excess salt is flushed out, the excess fluid goes with it. Another benefit of diuretics is that they help blood vessel walls to relax and widen, allowing the blood to pass through more easily and so lower blood pressure. Diuretics include bendroflumethiazide, chlortalidone, cyclopenthiazide, indapamide, metolazone, xipamide, bumetenide, furosemide, torasemide, eplerenone, spironolactone, triamterene and amiloride.

As with all blood pressure medications, diuretics are normally side-effect free. It's possible, though, to experience the following:

- thirstiness
- an increased need to pass urine
- weakness, lethargy, nausea and/or faintness
- muscle cramps
- skin rash
- male impotence
- raised blood sugar levels
- raised uric acid levels, possibly leading to gout or kidney problems
- low levels of potassium in the body, possibly leading to a dangerous condition called *hypokalaemia*.

As diuretics make you produce more urine than normal, you should take yours in the morning rather than late in the day when your sleep may be disturbed. You may require frequent blood and urine checks to ensure that your potassium, uric acid and sugar levels are normal.

Diuretics are long-term medications, just like all the blood pressure drugs. If you experience side effects or think you don't need to take diuretics any more, it's important that you speak to your doctor.

Taking blood pressure medication

Here are some suggestions for getting the most from your medication:

- Accept that you need to take blood pressure medication to protect your blood vessels and heart. Your body is unable to do this alone any more.
- Make your medicines a part of your daily routine, taking them at the same time every day. As your blood pressure is likely to be higher in the morning, it's best to take them with your breakfast.
- Read the information leaflets that come with your medication. If you are unsure of anything, ask your doctor.
- You may wish to monitor your blood pressure at home, between medical appointments. This will help you to see that your blood pressure medication is working. If it doesn't appear to be working, go back to your doctor.
- Remember that if you are able to lower your blood pressure by lifestyle changes, you will need to take less medication, or even stop it altogether.

8

Women and high blood pressure

If you are female and worried about high blood pressure in relation to contraception, pregnancy or after the menopause, you would be well advised to read this chapter.

Oestrogen

Oestrogen – commonly known as 'the female sex hormone' – is the name given to a group of chemicals that occur naturally in the female body. The main manufacturing site of oestrogen is the ovaries; however, a small amount is also produced by the adrenal glands, which sit on top of the kidneys. In pregnant women, the placenta (the organ in the womb that provides the developing child with nutrients) makes oestrogen, too.

Oestrogen is carried around the body in the bloodstream and affects cells in a variety of ways by attaching to them; the parts to which it attaches are known as *binding sites* or *receptors*. There are oestrogen receptors in your brain, bones, blood vessels and central nervous system. (The central nervous system comprises the brain and spinal cord. It is effectively the network of nerve tissues that controls the activities of the body.)

As oestrogen exerts a protective effect during a woman's reproductive years, she is less likely than a man to develop heart disease, stroke and so on. Levels of oestrogen rise during a girl's teenage years, controlling her reproductive system and allowing her to have babies. Its levels don't usually drop until during the menopause, when pregnancy is no longer an option. (See p. 111 for more information on oestrogen levels and the menopause.)

Here is a list of some of the important functions of oestrogen produced naturally:

- It is believed to affect the balance of cholesterol in the blood in a way that is beneficial, raising levels of 'good' HDL cholesterol and lowering levels of 'bad' LDL cholesterol. High levels of LDL cholesterol make a person more prone to developing blockage of the arteries (which often causes a heart attack), while HDL helps to prevent a blockage.

- As most strokes are caused by the same set of circumstances in the brain as can occur in the heart, oestrogen is thought to reduce the likelihood of stroke.
- Oestrogen helps to maintain the arteries and other blood vessels, possibly countering the tendency for some women to develop hardening of the arteries.
- There is evidence to suggest that oestrogen may protect a woman from developing Alzheimer's disease.
- Oestrogen keeps a woman's bones healthy and strong. During and after the menopause, women make far less of this group of hormones naturally, meaning that oestrogen deficiency is one of the main causes of bone loss.
- As there are even oestrogen receptors in a woman's skin, it is protected from drying and becoming thinner during her reproductive years. During and after the menopause, however, she is more likely to experience thinning skin that is prone to wrinkling.

As you can see from some of these points, the protective effect of oestrogen decreases as a woman grows older, and by the retirement years men and women share roughly the same degree of risk. Before the menopause a woman is less likely to develop high blood pressure, cardiovascular (heart) disease, stroke, and so on, than a man.

Oral contraceptives

A sexually active woman of reproductive age will, if she fails to use a good form of birth control, normally find herself getting pregnant at some point. One very effective birth control method is the combined oral contraceptive pill (known as the COCP) – often referred to as 'the birth-control pill' or simply 'the Pill' – which is a combination of synthetic female hormones developed specifically to prevent pregnancy. It is currently used by more than 100 million women worldwide and, in most cases, effectively prevents the female egg cell (technically termed the *ovum*) being released from one of the woman's two ovaries into the adjoining Fallopian tube, where it would otherwise be fertilized by her partner's sperm. The COCP has therefore prevented many unwanted pregnancies and allowed couples to plan their families.

Side effects

Although 50–60 per cent of women report no side effects from taking the COCP, others can experience such things as headaches, dizziness, blurred vision, nausea, weight gain, skin problems, vaginal discharge, reduced libido and changes in menstrual flow. There is one possible side effect that fails to create symptoms, however, and that is high blood pressure – a problem that is often undiscovered until something happens which requires medical attention. If you take the COCP or are considering taking it, make sure your doctor monitors your blood pressure on a regular basis. You can also reduce the risk of developing high blood pressure by carefully following the lifestyle advice in this book: a woman who takes the COCP and smokes is far more likely to develop cardiovascular disease or stroke, for example, than if she continues taking the COCP and quits smoking.

If you experience reduced libido (a fall in sexual desire) you would be best advised to get your blood pressure checked. Reduced libido can be an indicator of high blood pressure in some women.

Any woman taking the COCP should have her blood pressure monitored regularly. You can also check it yourself between visits to your health centre by the use of self-monitoring equipment (see Chapter 1). If you are having symptoms or your blood pressure is raised, your doctor may first want to try you with a different COCP – there are plenty of choices. For many of the women affected, however, high blood pressure will always be a problem when they take the COCP and they may be left with no choice but to discontinue its use. A woman who already has high blood pressure without using the COCP will not be offered a prescription for it by her doctor – using the COCP would be likely to increase her current health risks.

Studies have found that the COCP can increase a woman's risk for liver cancer – the chances of her developing this are normally very low. It was found that Caucasian (white) women in the United States and Europe who take the COCP are at greater risk of developing liver cancer than African and Asian women, particularly if they use this type of contraceptive for a prolonged length of time.

Pregnancy

In some women, blood pressure may also increase as a result of pregnancy, which can be dangerous for both the mother and her baby. Many babies born to mothers with high blood pressure are perfectly healthy, but the condition can cause low birth weight and premature delivery. The mother, on the other hand, can experience kidney damage and other organ impairment.

If you have high blood pressure and are considering getting pregnant, it's important that you discuss the matter with your doctor first of all. He or she can then help you to get your blood pressure under control before and during the pregnancy.

Prior to becoming pregnant

I would advise that you make determined efforts to avoid pregnancy until your blood pressure is under control. This will involve following the lifestyle advice in earlier pages, such as limiting the salt in your diet, stopping smoking, taking regular exercise, avoiding alcohol and eating a healthy diet. If you are overweight it will also help you if you drop to a more healthy weight for your height.

If you take medication to control your blood pressure, it's important that you ask your doctor what to do about taking it while you are pregnant. You may be able to continue taking it, or it may be a type that could possibly harm the unborn child, in which case the medication could be changed. It's always best, however, if you can control your blood pressure entirely by making the right lifestyle changes before becoming pregnant. There is always some concern about the effects of medications on an unborn child.

During the pregnancy

Antenatal (also called *prenatal*) health care is vital for women with a history of high blood pressure. It is also important for the remainder of pregnant women, as some develop high blood pressure for the first time at some point during the pregnancy and antenatal care will spot this. Although I had never previously been troubled by high blood pressure, my own blood pressure shot up during each of my three pregnancies. Indeed, it became so high that a syndrome known as *pre-eclampsia* developed.

Pre-eclampsia

Pre-eclampsia (sometimes known as *toxaemia of pregnancy*) is actually a combination of high blood pressure (measuring 140/90 or more on at least two separate readings) and raised levels of protein in the urine (300 mg in a 24-hour sample). This is a serious condition which occurs in as many as 10 per cent of pregnancies and can threaten the lives of both the mother and her unborn child, particularly if it develops as early as 20–32 weeks into the pregnancy. Blood pressure elevation is the most apparent sign of the disorder, but it also involves possible damage to the endothelium – the tissue forming the lining of cells and various organs in the body such as the blood vessels, lymphatic vessels and heart. The condition can also cause damage to the mother's kidneys and liver. The only known cure is pregnancy termination, early induction of labour to deliver the child or Caesarean section, again to deliver the child. In my own cases, there was no lasting damage; however, although my blood pressure returned to normal after my first two children were born, it remained high after the birth of my third child. High blood pressure runs in my family and I was only able to control it, and so stop taking medication, when I made the lifestyle changes described in this book.

I'm afraid that women who retain normal blood pressure for the duration of their pregnancy aren't quite out of the woods, either, once the child is delivered. Indeed, high blood pressure can develop up to six weeks after the birth and is the most common of postnatal complications.

Pre-eclampsia is more likely to occur in women with pre-existing high blood pressure, diabetes, renal disease or an autoimmune disease such as rheumatoid arthritis or lupus.

Fulminant pre-eclampsia and eclampsia

Pre-eclampsia will occasionally progress to the more severe *fulminant pre-eclampsia*, the symptoms of which include headaches, visual disturbances, pains in the part of the abdomen immediately over the stomach and the condition called *eclampsia*. In eclampsia, the woman experiences convulsions, often followed by a coma. This obviously poses a dire threat to both the mother and her developing child.

What causes pre-eclampsia?

Many experts believe that some cases of pre-eclampsia are caused by a shallowly implanted placenta which becomes deficient in oxygen. This is thought to lead to an immune system response which acts on the endothelium – the tissue lining the cells and various organs such as the blood vessels, lymphatic vessels and heart. The shallow implantation of the placenta in the lining of the womb is believed to stem from the woman's immune reaction. In other words, her body may lack the normal receptors to the proteins used by the placenta, and therefore her immune system sets up a destructive attack on the tissues of the developing foetus, causing her blood pressure and protein levels to rise and harm to come to the child – i.e. miscarriage or stillbirth. This opinion is consistent with evidence showing that miscarriages are often linked with an immunological disorder in the mother.

Where the placenta is allowed to implant normally – as happens in many cases – experts think that pre-eclampsia develops because the woman has a lowered tolerance for the inflammatory burden of pregnancy.

Gestational hypertension

Some pregnant women develop high blood pressure without the presence of protein in the urine. This is called *gestational hypertension* or *pregnancy-induced hypertension*. It is as serious a condition as pre-eclampsia and requires the same careful monitoring.

During and after the menopause

During and after the menopause, a woman's oestrogen levels decline dramatically. This significantly raises her chance of developing high blood pressure and its associated conditions.

Postmenopausal hormone replacement therapy

For a long time it was believed that, thanks to the beneficial effects of oestrogen on LDL cholesterol levels (see p. 105), hormone replacement therapy (HRT, which largely contains oestrogen) would prevent cardiovascular (heart) disease, stroke and so on. Some experts are still of this opinion. Indeed, there have been long-term 'observational' studies where women who were followed over time appeared to have a lower risk of developing high blood pressure and its associated disorders. However, such studies are classed as unreliable as they were not controlled enough to give definitive answers.

Thankfully, numerous controlled studies into the efficacy of HRT have since taken place – and they have produced a great body of evidence which strongly suggests that HRT does not have a protective effect and that actually it slightly increases a woman's chances of developing diseases related to high blood pressure. Unfortunately, too many doctors have not yet updated their opinion, and it can only be hoped that they will do so very soon.

Coping with menopause symptoms

It is the symptoms of the menopause that usually send a woman to her doctor for a prescription of HRT. Problems such as hot flushes, in which the body is suddenly consumed by the sensation of intense heat, accompanied by night-time sweating are often the most difficult to bear. Mood swings can be a real problem, too – and HRT usually succeeds in resolving these issues. The possibility of high blood pressure and its related disorders developing at some point is really not worth the immediate relief, however, and you would be best advised to control menopause symptoms by using more natural means. There are several books on the subject, as mentioned in 'Further reading' (p. 117), some of which will be available in your local library and some from high-street bookshops.

Because certain herbs were believed to help regulate oestrogen levels, they have become increasingly popular in the management of menopause symptoms. The herbs most commonly used are black cohosh, sage, dong quai, red clover, wild yam, ginseng and chaste tree. However, in a series of studies into the efficacy of black cohosh, ginseng and chaste tree, none had any effect on the study participants' symptoms. There are plenty of smaller studies that suggest benefits from taking herbs, but experts can always find fault with these studies if they look for them. For example, in one study that was agreed to be scientifically valid, it was found that the use of dong quai did not affect hormonal blood levels or the growth of endometrial cells which line the uterus. These are both major physical changes which occur during the menopause, and a herb used to alleviate symptoms would be expected to affect these things.

Sage may be the most reliable herb to use for treating hot flushes, as it is known to directly decrease the production of sweat. It is best bought as dried leaves from a herbalist and drunk as a tea (a herbal infusion) three times a day.

If you wish to try using herbs to cope with menopause symptoms, you would be best advised to consult with a qualified herbalist.

Useful addresses

UK-based organizations

Alcoholics Anonymous
PO Box 1
10 Toft Green
York Y01 7ND
Tel.: 01904 644026
National Helpline: 0845 769 7555
Website: www.alcoholics-anonymous.org.uk

Blood Pressure Association
60 Cranmer Terrace
London SW17 0QS
Tel.: 020 8772 4994
Blood Pressure Information Line: 0845 241 0989 (11 a.m. to 3 p.m., Monday to Friday)
Website: www.bpassoc.org.uk

The only UK-wide charity that focuses solely on tackling high blood pressure. Offers a range of information and support to help people take control of, or avoid, this condition.

British Heart Foundation
Greater London House
180 Hampstead Road
London NW1 7AW
Tel.: 020 7554 0000 (9 a.m. to 5 p.m, Monday to Friday)
Heart HelpLine: 0300 330 3311 (9 a.m. to 6 p.m., Monday to Friday)
Website: www.bhf.org.uk

Provides a range of information about the causes, prevention and treatment of heart disease. There is also a glossary and details of publications, plus practical advice on how to protect yourself from heart disease.

British Hypertension Society
Website: www.bhsoc.org

Provides a medical and scientific research forum to enable sharing of cutting-edge research, in order to understand the origin of high blood pressure and improve its treatment.

For professional enquiries about information on hypertension:
Jackie Howarth
BHS Administrative Officer
Clinical Sciences Building
Level 5
Leicester Royal Infirmary
PO Box 65
Leicester LE2 7LX
Tel.: 07717 467 973

For enquiries about meetings, membership etc.:
Mrs Gerry McCarthy
Meetings Secretary
Hampton Medical Conferences Ltd
113–119 High Street
Hampton Hill
Middlesex TW12 1NJ
Tel.: 020 8979 8300
Website: www.hamptonmedical.com

High Blood Pressure Foundation
Department of Medical Sciences
Western General Hospital
Edinburgh EH4 2XU
Tel.: 0131 332 9211
Website: www.hbpf.org.uk

Aims to improve the basic understanding, assessment, treatment and
public awareness of high blood pressure, and in so doing help promote
the welfare of people with the condition.

NHS Direct
Helpline: 0845 4647 (24 hours a day)
Website: www.nhsdirect.nhs.uk

This 24-hour NHS service provides expert health advice from trained
nurses. An extensive database of medical information is available on the
website. The nurses can also advise you if you wish to make a complaint
about the NHS.

NHS Smoking Helpline
Tel.: 0800 022 4332 (7 a.m. to 11 p.m., 7 days a week)
Website: www.nhs.uk/smokefree

A website giving support and advice on how to quit smoking, with
information on local-group sessions, a programme giving support at
home and advice on how nicotine replacement products can help you to
manage cravings.

QUIT
63 St Mary's Axe
London EC3A 8AA
Tel.: 0207 469 0400
Quitline: 0800 00 22 00 (for free, individual, same-day advice from
trained counsellors)
Website: www.quit.org.uk

The aim of QUIT is to significantly reduce unnecessary suffering and
death from smoking-related diseases. It provides practical help, advice and
support to smokers who wish to stop.

Sleep Matters
Tel.: 020 8994 9874 (6 p.m. to 8 p.m., 7 days a week)
Website: www.medicaladvisoryservice.org.uk/html/sleep_matters.html

A nurse-run information line operated by the Medical Advisory Service.
For help and advice on overcoming insomnia and achieving a good
night's sleep.

Stress Management Society
Tel.: 0844 357 8629
Website: www.stress.org.uk

A non-profit organization dedicated to helping people tackle stress.

The Stroke Association
Stroke House
240 City Road
London EC1V 2PR
Tel.: 020 7566 0300
Stroke Helpline: 0845 3033 100 (9 a.m. to 5 p.m., Monday to Friday)
Website: www.stroke.org.uk

Provides information and support for people affected by stroke.

Outside the UK

American Heart Association
National Center
7272 Greenville Avenue
Dallas, TX 75231
Tel.: 1 800 242 8721
Website: www.americanheart.org

For a wealth of information, tools and resources about cardiovascular
disease and stroke, to help you manage your health.

Blood Pressure Canada
Website: www.hypertension.ca

A web-based non-profit charitable organization dedicated to the prevention and control of hypertension (high blood pressure). Strives to increase awareness about the condition and reduce the burden of cardiovascular disease.

Further reading

Beevers, G., *Understanding Blood Pressure*. Family Doctor Publications, London, 2006.

Beevers, G., Lip, G. Y. H. and O'Brien, E., *ABC of Hypertension*. Wiley-Blackwell, Oxford, 2007.

Brewer, S., *Overcoming High Blood Pressure: The complete complementary health programme*. Duncan Baird, London, 2008.

Brewer, S. and Berriedale-Johnson, M., *Eat to Beat High Blood Pressure: Natural self-help for hypertension, including 60 recipes*. Thorsons, London, 2003.

Glenville, M., *New Natural Alternatives to HRT*. Kyle Cathie, London, 2003.

Kowalski, R. E., *8 Weeks to Lower Blood Pressure: Take the pressure off your heart without the use of prescription drugs*. Vermilion, London, 2007.

McKenna, P., *Quit Smoking Today without Gaining Weight* (book and CD). Bantam Press, London, 2007.

Marsh, G., *Hypertension: Exercise plans to reduce your blood pressure*. A. & C. Black, London, 2010.

Riley, R., *How to Stop Smoking and Stay Stopped for Good*. Vermilion, London, 2007.

Rubin, A. L., *High Blood Pressure for Dummies*. John Wiley & Sons, Chichester, 2007.

Smith, T., *Living with High Blood Pressure*. Sheldon Press, London, 2001.

Smith, T., *Living with Angina*. Sheldon Press, London, 2009.

Index